Measurement in Health Behavior

MEASUREMENT IN HEALTH BEHAVIOR

Methods for Research and Education

Colleen Konicki Di Iorio

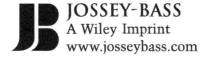

JOSSEY-BASS
A Wiley Imprint
www.josseybass.com

Published by Jossey-Bass
A Wiley Imprint
989 Market Street, San Francisco, CA 94103-1741   www.josseybass.com

Jossey-Bass books and products are available through most bookstores. To contact Jossey-Bass directly call our Customer Care Department within the U.S. at 800-956-7739, outside the U.S. at 317-572-3986, or fax 317-572-4002.

Jossey-Bass also publishes its books in a variety of electronic formats. Some content that appears in print may not be available in electronic books.

Library of Congress Cataloging-in-Publication Data
Di Iorio, Colleen Konicki, 1947-
  Measurement in health behavior : methods for research and education /
Colleen Konicki Di Iorio.
    p. ; cm.
  Includes bibliographical references and index.
  ISBN 978-0-7879-7097-0 (alk. paper)
  1. Health behavior--Measurement. 2. Health
behavior--Research--Methodology.
  [DNLM: 1. Health Behavior. 2. Data Collection. 3. Reproducibility of
Results. W 85 D575m 2005] I. Title.
  RA776.9.D54 2005
  362.1072--dc22
                        2005027390

FIRST EDITION
PB Printing 10 9 8 7 6 5 4 3 2

CONTENTS

TABLES, FIGURES, AND EXHIBITS

Tables

Figures

Exhibits

To the memory of my parents,
Thaddeus M. Konicki and Mary Hogan Konicki

PREFACE

This text is written primarily for public health students, particularly those in health education and health behavior programs. Students in other health disciplines, including nursing, medicine, applied health sciences, and psychology, may also find it useful. This book is intended to be an introductory text for students and public health professionals who have a limited background in statistics and mathematics, yet need a basic understanding of measurement issues. It emphasizes classical measurement strategies for constructing instruments, for testing for reliability and validity, and for interpreting results. A major portion of the text deals with scale development and testing, but chapters on survey development and the construction of knowledge tests are also included. Likewise, even though classical test theory is the major theoretical approach, generalizability theory and item response theory are also introduced.

The approach used stresses the practical application of concepts and principles. With that in mind, I have used data from research and programs that I have been involved in during the past ten years to provide realistic examples from public health that demonstrate the concepts. This book also includes illustrations of materials used to gather evaluative data, and instructions for conducting tests of reliability and validity using SPSS. Samples of SPSS printouts are provided, along with detailed interpretations of the results.

The overall objectives of this text are to improve the student's (1) knowledge of instrument development and testing using classical test theory, (2) understanding of reports of reliability and validity testing found in articles and reports, (3) ability to conduct basic tests for reliability and validity, and (4) ability to interpret the results of data analysis. To accomplish these aims, the book is divided into thirteen chapters. The first three chapters provide a background in measurement theory. In Chapter One, the definition of measurement is presented, along with a brief history of measurement in the psychological and health sciences and a discussion of the advantages of measurement. Chapter Two presents a brief description of the different types of measures that might be used to collect data about health behavior or factors associated with it. Chapter Three presents a discussion of the types of measurement error and strategies to reduce error.

Chapters Four and Five present overviews of survey development and knowledge test construction, respectively. Chapter Six begins a discussion of scale development, which is the focus for the remainder of the book. This chapter presents important information on the analysis of concepts. In Chapter Seven, the principles of item writing and of formatting summated rating scales are discussed. Chapter Eight presents basic statistical concepts that are necessary for understanding the material in the following chapters. Chapters Nine and Ten focus on reliability: Chapter Nine discusses classical test theory, and Chapter Ten examines the different types of reliability assessment. The final three chapters of the book focus on validity testing. In Chapter Eleven, the concept of validity is introduced and several strategies for assessing validity are discussed. In Chapter Twelve, the basic principles of factor analysis are presented. The final chapter, Chapter Thirteen, provides an elementary description of item response theory.

Examples and data analyses described in several of the chapters rely heavily on my research in HIV prevention and self-management of chronic illnesses. This work has been supported by several agencies including the National Institute of Mental Health, the National Institute of Nursing Research, the National Institute of Child Health and Human Development, the Centers for Disease Control and Prevention, the Epilepsy Foundation, and the Emory University Research Committee.

Acknowledgments

There are many people who have helped bring this book to completion. First are the students in my classes at the Rollins School of Public Health, who provided the inspiration for the book. I especially want to thank the students in the measurement classes of spring 2004 and spring 2005. These students used drafts of the book for their class text and provided invaluable feedback on the content and the presentation, for which I am grateful. I also want to thank Amanda Whatley and Andrea Landis, who critiqued each chapter from a student's perspective and provided comments to improve the clarity of the text. Many thanks also to those who read drafts of the book and provided feedback, especially Stanley A. Mulaik, Frances McCarty, Ronda Sinkowitz-Cochran, and Amy Lansky. I am indebted to Stanley Mulaik who provided many helpful comments throughout the book, in particular on reliability assessment and factor analysis. His perspective on the use of factor analysis for instrument development is clearly evident in Chapter Twelve. Frances McCarty combed the chapters and recommended a number of changes that helped clarify difficult concepts. She also contributed to the section on analysis of variance and wrote the final chapter on item response theory. Ronda Sinkowitz-Cochran and Amy Lansky reviewed the chapters from the practitioner's perspective, and their suggestions for revisions improved the link between theory and practice. I appreciate the support of those who helped with the compilation of the book, and I especially want to thank Pamela Kennedy, Regina Daniel, and Sara Di Iorio for their many hours of assistance with gathering references, formatting chapters, and other tasks. Not forgotten are the many students who made numerous trips to the library for materials.

I am also indebted to my family for their patience and support. Special thanks go to my husband, Ralph; my children, Matt and Sara; and my sisters, Susan Arrowood, Doris Konicki, Mary Morin, Carol Konicki, Nancy Konicki, and Pamela Kennedy.

August 2005   Colleen Konicki Di Iorio
Atlanta, Georgia

THE AUTHOR

Colleen Konicki Di Iorio is a professor in the Department of Behavioral Sciences and Health Education at Rollins School of Public Health and holds a secondary appointment in the Department of Family and Community Nursing at the Nell Hodgson Woodruff School of Nursing. She earned her Ph.D. degree in nursing research and theory development from New York University, her master's degree in nursing from New York University, and her bachelor's degree in nursing from the University of Iowa. She is a registered nurse and a Fellow of the American Academy of Nursing. She has extensive experience in health promotion research and instrument development. Her research on health behavior has been funded by the Centers for Disease Control and Prevention, the National Institutes of Health, and the Epilepsy Foundation, among others. Her work focuses on two broad areas of health: adherence and self-management, and HIV prevention. Di Iorio has published widely in the health behavior literature. She has served as a consultant to and been a member of panels of professional and community organizations and governmental agencies. She currently serves as the associate editor of the *Journal of Nursing Measurement*. She recently received the Distinguished Nurse Scholar Award from New York University and the Distinguished Alumni Award from the University of Iowa.

Measurement in Health Behavior

CHAPTER ONE

INTRODUCTION TO MEASUREMENT

LEARNING OBJECTIVES

At the end of this chapter, the student should be able to

1. Give two reasons for taking a measurement course.
2. Describe major historical events in the development of measurement theory.
3. List three measurement skills that public health students can use in their careers.
4. Define the term *measurement*.
5. List four advantages of measurement.
6. Compare and contrast the four levels of measurement.
7. Define the terms *reliability* and *validity*.

Role of Measurement in Health Education and Health Behavior Research

Public health students are often surprised to learn that measurement of health behaviors requires special study. Students often associate measurement theory with research and sometimes question its applicability to the everyday work of health professionals. Yet a close examination of the work of health professionals reveals the pervasiveness of measurement issues. Consider, for example, Nelini, who is employed as a health educator by a large public hospital. Nelini develops and conducts self-management classes for adults with epilepsy. She knows that the people who attend the classes enjoy them, because they tell her so. But the hospital is faced with budget cuts, and the hospital administrator has asked Nelini and others to justify the existence of their programs. Nelini knows that a successful program would make the people who attend her classes more comfortable and confident in dealing with issues that surround living with epilepsy and would encourage them to take their medications on a regular basis. They might have fewer seizures or fewer side effects of seizures as a result of taking their medications properly and living a healthy life. To demonstrate that her program is effective, Nelini must evaluate it. This evaluation is likely to include a survey measuring self-management skills and important outcomes associated with self-management.

Other graduates of health education and behavioral sciences programs have similar experiences. Take Sara, a new graduate with a master's degree in public health (MPH) hired recently by a large research firm. In the few short months since she started working for the company, her assignments have varied, and some involve an understanding of measurement. For instance, she recently consulted with a group of researchers in California on how to use focus groups to generate items for a research questionnaire on smoking behaviors of middle school adolescents. She assisted in the development of the focus group interview guide and the writing of items for the questionnaire; both tasks required an understanding of measurement principles.

Matt works at a university school of public health as the project director of a federally funded study. The purpose of the study is to evaluate an intervention designed to increase physical activity among older men and women. Matt's responsibilities include locating self-report measures of exercise and physical activity appropriate for people over sixty-five years of age who live in both urban and rural areas, and assessing the feasibility of those measures for the current study. Matt must also locate biobehavioral measures of strength and endurance that will be used to augment the self-report measures. During the course of the study, Matt will be involved in the preliminary studies to assess the psychometric properties of the instruments to be used in it. While the main study is conducted, he will monitor the collection of data using the measures and ensure that the data are collected according to protocol.

Rao, a graduate of an MPH program with an emphasis in global health, is also applying his knowledge of measurement, as a member of the HIV task force in India. Street youth attend the HIV prevention program he has developed; classes are held in an open field next to a temple. During the past year, he has expanded the program to include other services such as vocational and literacy training. Currently, Rao is attempting to locate additional funding for these new programs, and potential funding agencies have requested information about the effectiveness of the programs. Rao's task is to decide what outcomes of the program are important to measure and how to measure them. In conducting an assessment of outcomes, he faces special challenges because the children neither read nor write and cultural differences preclude the use of questionnaires or interviews developed for other populations.

These examples highlight the variety of measurement skills used by public health professionals. They also demonstrate the importance of exposure to measurement issues in training programs, which creates an advantage for students when they take on work assignments. In summary, then, a course in measurement can introduce students in public health to the basic principles of measurement, including concept analysis, item writing and analysis, data collection procedures, and assessment of measures for use in research or evaluation studies.

Brief History of Psychosocial Measurement

The history of measurement dates back to the first man or woman who devised a system to count objects. Unfortunately, we do not know how or why this conceptual leap occurred, but it defined a monumental transition point in human history. Over time, people invented procedures to measure length and weight, and fields of study (for example, astronomy and physics) evolved that required various forms of measurement. Theories of measurement and quantity were also proposed by philosophers and mathematicians, including Aristotle and Euclid (Michell, 1990). The study and assessment of human capabilities have a long history as well. No doubt our early ancestors devised methods to evaluate and reward physical characteristics that were important in everyday and military life. In ancient Greece, for example, the Olympic Games celebrated athletic achievements in human endurance and strength through public competition (Crane, 2004).

Recorded history of the measurement of human capabilities, however, can be traced back only 3,000 years, to ancient China. In the second century B.C., China used a system of examinations to assess eligibility for government positions and for retention and promotion in those positions. (See DuBois, 1970, for a detailed discussion of the history of psychological testing. Major events addressed in that book are described here.) Early examinations included assessments of archery, music, and writing; later ones assessed civil law, military affairs, and geography. This system of examinations, with modifications, continued in China until the early twentieth century. Great Britain adopted a similar system of examinations for government employees in the 1830s, and by the end of the nineteenth century, the U.S. Congress had established competitive testing for entry into government service in the United States.

Though China is credited with initiating testing for government employees, European universities and schools were the first to implement testing as a means of evaluating student learning. The earliest testing seems to have occurred in the Middle Ages, with the earliest formal examinations in 1219 at the University of Bologna

(DuBois, 1970). Teachers conducted oral examinations until the introduction of paper, after which written examinations predominated. Schools and universities in the American colonies adopted student testing as a means of assessing student learning and eligibility for degrees, and this testing continues today in most U.S. educational institutions.

Whereas today's civil service and academic examinations provide a foundation for the measurement of knowledge and professional skills, the work of European and American psychologists in the late nineteenth century furthered the study of measurement of individual differences, attitudes, and behaviors. Two British citizens, Sir Francis Galton and Karl Pearson, were among the first to work in the area of psychometric testing. Galton introduced the study of human differences in psychological functioning, the basic understanding of correlation between variables, and the development of the questionnaire for psychological research (DuBois, 1970). Pearson expanded Galton's work on correlation and developed the product moment correlation along with the chi-square goodness-of-fit test to examine the relationships between variables.

The initial work in the area of psychological measurement focused on individual differences in tests of motor and sensory functioning. These tests included reaction times for identifying sounds and naming colors, identification of least noticeable differences in weight, and tactile perception of touch and pain. The field of psychology experienced a dramatic shift in the late nineteenth century with the work of Alfred Binet (Binet & Simon, 1973). Binet recognized that tests involving complex mental processes might be more useful than the usual motor and sensory tests in distinguishing the important characteristics of individuals. His work focused on the development of tests to measure psychological processes such as memory, problem solving, judgment, and comprehension. Through careful testing, he established that success on the tests varied with the age of a child, the child's school year, and even his or her class standing as determined by the teacher. In 1905, Binet and Simon introduced the first intelligence test, which was a composite of individual tests. Used to develop norms for different age groups of children and for adults, and used widely in clinical evaluations, these early forays into more complicated testing inspired the development of other forms of mental assessment.

By the time the United States entered World War I, in 1917, a number of psychological tests were available, and psychologists expressed an interest in assisting in the evaluation of recruits. Robert Yerkes served as chairperson of the Psychology Committee of the National Research Council, whose primary objective was the psychological assessment of U.S. Army recruits (DuBois, 1970). Because of the overwhelming task of conducting individual assessments for all recruits, the committee decided to develop a group test. Their efforts resulted in the Army Alpha, the first psychological test administered on a large-scale basis using a group format. The Army used the assessment throughout the war, and by the end of the fighting, the testing program had opened a new avenue for the administration of tests and had expanded psychological testing into other areas. Interestingly, the Army Alpha used multiple-choice items, the success of which led to the adoption of multiple-choice items among educational measurement specialists.

In addition to measures of intelligence, psychologists developed measures of other psychological qualities. In the first quarter of the twentieth century, E. L. Thorndike, a noted educational measurement specialist, studied the interests and perceived abilities of students in academic subjects. (See, for example, Thorndike, 1913, 1920.) His work is particularly interesting because these measures incorporated ratings of degree of interest or perceived abilities. In 1922, Freyd published a paper describing the study of vocational interests. To assess interests in a variety of occupations, Freyd used a five-point response scale (*L!, L, ?, D, D!*) in which *L* represented *like* and *D* represented *dislike*. In 1923, Freyd described a type of graphic rating scale that came to be known as a visual analog scale. Other tests measured skills, aptitudes, and personality traits such as neuroticism, creativity, introversion/extroversion, and anxiety. Approaches to the development of scales were devised by several individuals including Thurstone (1925), Likert (1932), and Guttman (1944). These measures and others like them formed the basis for the later development and assessment of instruments designed to measure health behaviors.

The study of measures themselves was also a major research focus during the twentieth century. In the early 1900s, Spearman (1904) introduced the concept of *reliability* to refer to the consistency of a measure. Later he developed a procedure to compute the internal consistency of a measure and coined the term *reliability coefficient* (Spearman, 1910). Through the use of correlation, investigators were able to compare new measures to selected criteria or other, related concepts. In 1937, Kuder and Richardson published a method for calculating the internal-consistency reliability of dichotomous measures, and in 1951, Cronbach, building on their work and that of Spearman (1910) and Brown (1910), devised a general method for calculating internal consistency.

Advances in computer technology enabled significant advances to be made in psychometrics in the latter half of the twentieth century. Although researchers developed the basic ideas and calculations for complex techniques such as factor analysis and multidimensional scaling in the early part of the century, personnel and time demands hindered widespread use of these techniques. With the advent of personal computers and the software for them, researchers began to use these and other techniques in the assessment of instruments, further advancing the understanding of instrument development and testing.

In addition to developments in the availability of computers, advances were made in the theoretical approaches to instrument development and testing. The most important contributions were confirmatory factor analysis using structural equation modeling (SEM) (Jöreskog, 1969; James, Mulaik, & Brett, 1982), item response theory (IRT)

(Lord, 1953), and generalizability theory (G theory) (Cronbach, Rajaratnam, & Gleser, 1963). Before 1950, classical test theory (CTT) constituted the basis of instrument development and testing. Though useful, this approach proved inadequate to solve some complex measurement problems. Therefore, alternative approaches to the conceptualization of measurement, along with new evaluation techniques, evolved during the latter part of the century. These newer ideas and techniques are referred to as modern test theory.

Conceptualization of Measurement

As noted earlier, the study of measurement and quantity has a long history, which dates back to Aristotle (Michell, 1990). Until the 1930s, ideas about measurement that had been developed over time were applied to psychological measurement. However, in 1932, the British Association for the Advancement of Science formed a committee to examine psychophysical measurement. And according to Michell (1990), that inquiry precipitated the development of new approaches to understanding psychological measurement, though some of them were not very useful for psychology. S. S. Stevens (1946) proposed one conceptualization of measurement. And although Michell sharply criticizes Stevens's conceptualization, Stevens's ideas have been used extensively in understanding psychological measurement for the past fifty years. Because Stevens's view is so pervasive, the following discussion on measurement is based on his work. The interested student is encouraged to read Michell (1990) for alternative views on the conceptualization of measurement.

A good place to begin the study of measurement is to define the term *measurement*. Stevens (1946) proposed that measurement is the "assignment of numerals to objects or events according to rule." He later modified his definition to this one: "[M]easurement is the assignment of numerals to aspects of objects or events according to rule[s]" (Stevens, 1959, p. 24). This qualification of measurement was important, because it states that measurement applies to the attributes (properties) of objects rather than to the objects themselves. Limiting the application of measurement to objects alone allows only the counting of objects—for example, determining the number of people in a room. But applying measurement to attributes of objects allows the measurement of numerous properties—such as length, height, and weight. In public health the objects most often studied are people, communities, and systems. So aspects of these objects might include, for people, illnesses, health behaviors, and attitudes; for communities, size, location (urban or rural), air quality, and cultural norms; and for systems, system access (for example, access to care), policies, cost, and quality.

Using rules to assign numbers to attributes of objects implies that the process of assignment must be standardized and clear. The rules for using common measuring devices such as tape measures, bathroom scales, and thermometers are generally clear.

However, instruments measuring constructs such as access to care, quality of life, and health status may be accompanied by more complex administration and scoring procedures. In these cases an explicit statement of the rules is necessary to ensure accurate measurement of the attributes.

Lastly, inherent in the definition of measurement is the notion of quantification. Numbers are assigned to an attribute in such a way as to represent quantities of that attribute (Nunnally & Bernstein, 1994). Quantification of an attribute is necessary. By converting abstract concepts to the numerical system through the process of measurement, we create the capacity to perform mathematical and statistical operations. For example, although we can see the heights of two young children, we cannot determine whether one of them is taller than the other unless there is a markedly visible difference in their heights or they are standing side by side. If the children live in different countries and are similar in height, how can we determine which of them is taller? Converting the concept of height into a number allows us to quantify the height of the child in country A and compare his or her height to that of the child in country B.

By converting concepts to numbers, we can perform other mathematical functions as well. We can measure the height, calculate the body mass index, and determine the developmental stage for each child. We can then compare these aspects to the norms for the child's age group. We can also compute averages for groups and norms for age groups. Without the process of measurement, we would be forced to use a conceptual system to discuss the attributes of the children, thus limiting our statements to broad conceptual comparisons. We could say that the children are large or small, are short or tall, or develop slowly or quickly. We could say that one child appears to have more body fat than another, but we would be unable to give more precise comparisons such as the exact difference in body mass and its impact on health.

Figure 1.1 is a visual representation of the conversion of concepts to numbers. The model shows that the conversion occurs through a process of measurement and that error is associated with this process. As you read this book, you will learn about different types of measurement processes, errors of measurement associated with them, and strategies used to identify and reduce error.

FIGURE 1.1. CONCEPTUALIZATION OF THE MEASUREMENT PROCESS.

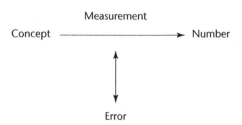

Reasons for Measuring Concepts

Assigning numbers that represent quantity to concepts allows us to perform operations related to the concepts that would be impossible without the conversions. For example, if we moved into a new apartment and wanted to purchase a table for the
dining room, how would we know the size of the table to buy? We could go to the store
and look for tables that seemed about the right size. But a better alternative would
be to measure the size of the room, to allow space to walk and to move the chairs
around the table, and from those figures to estimate the maximum size of an appropriate table for the room. Or we could go to the store, measure a table we liked, and
then go home and measure the size of the area to see whether the table would fit. The
point is that because we are able to measure the attributes of length and width, we can
determine, without actually bringing the table home, whether it will fit the assigned
space. Measurement, then, creates *flexibility*. It also allows us to compare similar concepts (for example, the length of the table and the length of the room) and to make
judgments about things without actually seeing them (for example, the fact that a table
10 feet long is larger than one that is 3 feet long).

The benefits of measurement also inform the daily work of health practice. A health
educator who wants to determine the success of a seminar for people with hypertension
can develop a test to evaluate changes in the participants' knowledge of hypertension. Rather than assume that participants have learned certain facts about hypertension,
the health educator can determine how many participants have understood the information by administering a test as an objective measure of this knowledge. Using the information gained from the test results, the health educator can determine how many items
participants answered correctly, thus quantifying the results. Using statistical tests,
the posttest results can be compared to the pretest results to determine the amount of
change in knowledge that can be attributed to the seminar. The health educator can evaluate the total scores on the test as well as on individual items to determine whether participants have learned some facts but not others. The information, in turn, is useful for
the improvement of the seminar or the *communication* of the results of the program to others. For example, the health educator can share the results with the participants or with
the funding agency. Once developed the test is available for every seminar, thus saving the
time and expense that would be involved in creating new methods of assessment for each
seminar. The health educator can compare the results over time to determine whether
the program is meeting its objectives. The test itself can be shared with other health
educators, thus increasing the ability to compare the effectiveness of different types of
hypertension programs in improving knowledge.

Measurement also provides the means by which we can test propositions from theory. In the present example, the health educator might have based the program on a

theory of behavioral change such as social cognitive theory, and thus might propose that participants who report higher levels of self-efficacy would also report higher rates of behavioral change. The health educator also might propose that participants in the seminar would be more likely to adopt strategies to control hypertension than partic- ipants in a control group. Using data collected from the pretests and posttests, the health educator could answer the research questions or test the hypotheses. The re- sults of these tests could determine whether or not the hypotheses were supported, which, in turn, could provide support (or not) for the theory itself.

Scales of Measurement

Another introductory concept that is important to the conceptualization of measure- ment proposed by Stevens is the categorization of measurement scales, also called levels of measurement. Stevens (1946) proposed that one can classify measurement scales according to the kind of transformations they can undergo without losing their properties. The four scale types he originally proposed are *nominal, ordinal, interval,* and *ratio;* the four properties of the scales, respectively, are *kind, order, equal intervals,* and *ratios* of individual values. Each scale can be transformed, but the transformations must main- tain the properties of the scale. Stevens refers to this characteristic as *invariance:* that is, the scale must retain its properties following transformation. Nominal scales are the least restrictive and can undergo a variety of transformations while maintaining their properties, whereas ratio scales are the most restrictive and can undergo few transfor- mations without changes in their properties. Because scale properties and their trans- formations are often confusing for students, we present a detailed description of each scale type, along with examples of measures used in health behavior research.

Nominal Scale

Nominal scales are used to classify variables that we can place in categories based on equivalence. Of the four scale properties listed above, the nominal-level variable is char- acterized by *kind.* More specifically, the categories of nominal-level variables differ in kind only. In regard to the other three properties of scales, nominal scales have no mean- ingful order such that assignment to one category indicates a greater or smaller amount of the variable. Likewise, the intervals between numbers on the scale are not equiva- lent, nor are ratios of individual values meaningful. An example of a nominal variable is the variable *gender* (also referred to as *sex).* It is composed of two categories: *male* and *female.* People are classified as either male or female, and all members of one group (for example, female) are the same on the variable (gender) but different from the members of the other group (male). Marital status is another common variable measured on the nominal scale. Although there are several possible categories of marital status, for this example we use the following: *married, never married, separated, widowed,* and *divorced.* People placed together in one of these categories have the same marital status, but differ on the marital status variable from people placed in the other categories.

The categories of a nominal scale must be mutually exclusive, meaning that a person, case, or event can be assigned to only one of the categories. The categories must also be exhaustive, so that all instances of an event or all of its characteristics can be categorized. If a researcher were interested in knowing how many of his or her participants were living with partners but not married, the marital status classification just discussed would fail to work. The researcher might elect to add another category, *living with a partner.* Adding this category would lead to overlapping categories, violating the principle that the categories must be mutually exclusive. A participant who has never been married but is living with a partner would be able to check two boxes, as would one who is divorced and living with a partner. In such a case, the researcher must determine exactly what information is important and develop categories that are both mutually exclusive and exhaustive.

Because the categories on a nominal scale differ only in kind and not in degree or amount, we can assign any number to each category as long as we use a different number for each. We could code male as 0 and female as 1 or vice versa. Because the particular numbers, and therefore any mathematical or statistical manipulation of the numbers, have no meaning, we could code male as 1003 and female as 62. By convention, though, the numbers 0 and 1 or 1 and 2 are used for coding the categories of gender. Nominal scales are the least restrictive in regard to the invariant criterion because no matter what numbers we choose, the property of the scale that categories differ in kind remains unchanged. The other properties of scales do not apply to nominal-level variables. That is, nominal-level variables have no meaningful order that would lead us to consider that a male has more gender than a female or vice versa.

The literature contains some controversy about whether classification as employed in the nominal scale is a true form of measurement (Lord & Novick, 1968; Stevens, 1959). Recall that we said that numbers are assigned to represent quantities of attributes. With nominal level scales, assigned numbers do not represent quantity, a seeming violation of the definition of measurement. Stevens (1959) contends that classification is a form of measurement because the assignment of numbers is done according to the rule of not assigning the same number to different categories or different numbers to the same category. Nunnally and Bernstein (1994, p. 1) provide a more refined definition of measurement that addresses this issue directly: "Measurement consists of rules for assigning symbols to objects so as to (1) represent quantities of attributes numerically (scaling) or (2) define whether the objects fall in the same or different categories with respect to a given attribute (classification)." Thus, nominal level variables meet the conditions for the second definition of measurement.

Ordinal Scale

Variables measured on an ordinal scale are those whose categories have a meaningful order that is *hierarchical* in nature. For example, the variable *college standing*, with the categories of *freshman, sophomore, junior,* and *senior,* is an ordinal variable. The categories represent an increasing number of credit hours completed; *freshman* represents the smallest number of credit hours and *senior* represents the largest. An important point to note, however, is that there is likely to be variability in the attributes within the categories. Thus, the category of *freshman* might include students who are just beginning their college careers and have not completed any coursework as well as those who have completed the maximum of credit hours for freshmen. Likewise, sophomores include those whose numbers of credit hours range from the least to the most for that classification. The grade of heart murmurs is another ordinal variable. Heart murmurs are graded from 1 to 6 depending on their severity. The variable is ordinal because there are higher levels of cardiac dysfunction as the grade of the murmur increases from 1 to 6. The numbers 1 through 6 indicate increasing severity in the heart murmur, but do not reflect the actual amount of increased severity.

Rating scales that use responses such as *strongly agree, agree, neither agree nor disagree, disagree,* and *strongly disagree* are considered ordinal scales. The categories of such a scale are distinct and differ in degree. The categories are ordered so that a report of *agree* suggests a more favorable attitude than that of *disagree.* However, there is likely a range of feelings among people responding in each category. For those who respond *agree,* some may lean more toward *strongly agree* and others may be closer to *neither agree nor disagree.* The numbers assigned to the categories can only reflect the order of the categories. The numbers cannot represent the precise degrees of difference in attitude between the categories.

Variables measured on an ordinal scale will remain unchanged under transformations in which the order of the categories is always maintained. Transformations include adding a constant to all the numbers or multiplying the numbers by a constant. Thus we could code college class status as 1, 2, 3, and 4 to represent the four classes from *freshman* to *senior.* The numbers selected must always reflect the order. Thus, if we are using these numbers, freshmen must always be coded as 1 and seniors must always be coded as 4. But as shown in Exhibit 1.1, if we added 18 to each of the numbers or multiplied each

EXHIBIT 1.1. TRANSFORMATION OF AN ORDINAL VARIABLE BY ADDITION AND BY MULTIPLICATION.

(1 + 18), (2 + 18), (3 + 18), (4 + 18) = 19, 20, 21, 22

(1 x 44), (2 x 44), (3 x 44), (4 x 44) = 44, 88, 132, 176

number by 44, the actual numbers would change, but the rank order of the numbers would remain the same. Thus, any transformation that maintains this original order is acceptable.

Interval Scale

Variables measured on the interval scale have a *meaningful order:* higher levels have more of the attribute. Unlike those of the nominal and ordinal scales, the numbers used to represent the attribute measured on an interval scale are themselves meaningful and provide information about the amount of the attribute. In addition, interval scales have equal intervals, so that the distances between the successive units of measure are equivalent. The interval scale does not have a true zero point, a point at which there is nothing left of the attribute. Without the true zero point, the interpretation of ratios of individual values on the scale is not meaningful. However, the interpretation of ratios of differences is still meaningful. This concept is usually confusing for students, so we will give two examples to explain it.

The most common example of an interval scale is temperature measured in degrees Fahrenheit. A temperature of 100 degrees Fahrenheit is greater than one of 60 degrees Fahrenheit. Moreover, all the degrees of heat (molecular activity) are equivalent. Thus the difference in the amount of heat between 100 degrees and 60 degrees (40 degrees) is equivalent to the difference between 30 degrees and 70 degrees (40 degrees). We can also say that the difference in the amount of heat between 100 degrees and 60 degrees (40 degrees) is twice that of the difference between 50 degrees and 30 degrees (20 degrees) (ratios of differences). We cannot say, however, that 60 degrees is twice as hot as 30 degrees (ratio of individual values).

For a second example, suppose a researcher knows that the average birth weight for a particular group of infants is 7 pounds. The researcher wants to determine how much each infant deviates from the average weight. If the researcher recalibrated the scale with the mean weight set at 0, then 7 pounds would be coded as 0 (Figure 1.2). A baby weighing 8 pounds would receive a score of +1; a baby weighing 9 pounds, a score of +2; and so on. A baby weighing 6 pounds would receive a score of −1; one weighing 5 pounds, a score of −2. Using the new interval scale, as shown in Figure 1.2, we could say that the difference in weight between −2 and 0 (2 pounds) is equivalent to the difference in weight between +2 and +4 (2 pounds). However, we could not say that a baby with a score of +4 (11 pounds) weighs twice as much as one with a score of +2 (9 pounds).

When a scale has an arbitrary zero point, we can transform the scale by adding or multiplying by a constant. Thus, subtracting 32 from a Fahrenheit temperature and then multiplying the result by $\frac{5}{9}$ will change the scale from Fahrenheit degrees to Celsius degrees. Exhibit 1.2 shows the conversion of the Fahrenheit temperatures mentioned previously to Celsius temperatures. Note that when the Fahrenheit temperatures

FIGURE 1.2. INTERVAL SCALE FOR WEIGHTS OF NEWBORNS USING THE MEAN WEIGHT AS THE ORIGIN.

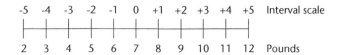

are converted to Celsius, the differences between the high and low temperatures in the two examples are equivalent (for example, 22 degrees). That is, the difference between 37.4°C and 15.4°C is equal to the difference between 20.9°C and –1.1°C. However, on the Fahrenheit scale, 60 degrees is twice 30 degrees, whereas the same temperature measured in Celsius—15.4°C—is not twice as much as –1.1°C. Thus, the interpretation of the ratios of individual values is not invariant when temperatures are converted from Fahrenheit to Celsius degrees.

An interval scale is considered to have an underlying continuous measure, whereas categories of variables measured on the ordinal scale are separated into distinct groups (for example, *freshman, sophomore, junior,* and *senior*). Although it is possible to convert interval-level variables into categories, the interpretation of the categories must take into

EXHIBIT 1.2. CONVERSION OF TEMPERATURE FROM FAHRENHEIT TO CELSIUS DEGREES.

Proof showing ratios of differences are equivalent:

$$\frac{5}{9}(°F - 32) = °C$$

$\frac{5}{9}(100°F - 32) = 37.7°C$	$\frac{5}{9}(70°F - 32) = 21.1°C$
$\frac{5}{9}(60°F - 32) = 15.5°C$	$\frac{5}{9}(30°F - 32) = -1.1°C$
Differences: 40°F 22.2°C	Differences: 40°F 22.2°C

100°F – 60°F is equivalent to 70°F – 30°F (both are 40°F).
37.7°C – 15.5°C is equivalent to 21.1°C – (–1.1)°C (both are 22.2°C).

Proof showing ratios of individual values are not equivalent:

The ratio $\frac{60}{100}$ is not equivalent to $\frac{15.5}{37.7}$.   The ratio $\frac{30}{70}$ is not equivalent to $\frac{-1.1}{21.1}$.

account the context of the conversion. Any attempt to categorize temperatures as low, medium, or high (ordinal scale) would depend on the situation. Categories of low, medium, and high for the temperature of the human body would differ from low, medium, and high air temperatures. Another consideration is that although we might report temperature in whole numbers, we can also measure temperature to a fraction of a degree. In some situations, it might make sense to measure temperature to the tenth or one-hundredth of a degree. The continuous scale allows these fine distinctions, whereas an ordinal scale does not.

As we have implied above, because an interval scale has an arbitrary zero point, negative values represent actual amounts of the attribute and thus have meaning. We know that Fahrenheit temperature is a measure of heat. Because 0 degrees is an arbitrary number, at 0 degrees Fahrenheit there is still molecular activity (heat) that can be measured. Indeed, air temperatures as low as –50 degrees Fahrenheit have been recorded. Likewise, when the researcher codes infant weights using the average weight as the zero point, a score of –3 is associated with an actual value of weight and has meaning.

Ratio Scale

The ratio scale has all the characteristics of the interval scale except for the arbitrary zero point. A ratio scale has a true zero point, a point at which nothing is left of the attribute. The true zero point permits the *meaningful expression of ratios*. Thus, as with an interval scale, we can say that the difference between 2 and 4 is the same as the difference between 4 and 6 (ratio of differences). However—and this is not the case with an interval scale—we can also say that 8 is twice as much as 4 (ratio of individual values). Both height and weight are measured on a ratio scale. Nothing is left to measure when height or weight is 0. A person with a blood pressure of 0 will not live long without medical intervention. Likewise, molecules do not move and generate heat where the Fahrenheit temperature is –460 (0 Kelvin, or absolute temperature). Because the measure of weight has a true zero point, a baby weighing 10 pounds is twice as heavy as one weighing 5 pounds.

Ratio scales have more restrictions on the types of transformations that can be applied, and they remain invariant only when values are multiplied by a constant. Thus, multiplying weight in pounds by 16 (the number of ounces in a pound) will convert 10 pounds to 160 ounces. When measured in ounces rather than pounds, the difference between the weights of a baby weighing 80 ounces and one weighing 160 ounces is the same as the difference between the weights of a baby weighing 112 ounces and one weighing 192 ounces. Likewise, after the conversion of weight from pounds to ounces, a baby who weighs 160 ounces remains twice as heavy as a baby who weighs 80 ounces.

A useful schema of the differences among the four measurement scales is shown in Figure 1.3.

FIGURE 1.3. SCHEMA FOR LEVELS OF MEASUREMENT.

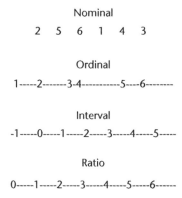

Nominal

2   5   6   1   4   3

Ordinal

1-----2-------3-4-----------5----6--------

Interval

-1-----0-----1-----2-----3-----4-----5-----

Ratio

0-----1-----2-----3-----4-----5-----6------

Levels of Measurement and Statistics

Stevens (1959) extended his classification of variables to include allowable statistical operations for each level of measurement. In general, an inverse relationship exists between allowable transformations and allowable statistics. The variables with the fewest restrictions on transformation (nominal scale) have the most restrictions in terms of statistical operations. Thus, if a data set included only variables measured on the nominal scale, the number of possible statistical tests would be limited. Frequencies and percentages could describe single variables, and we could use the mode as the measure of central tendency. However, significance tests would be limited to the chi-square or a similar statistic. For example, we could calculate the number and percentage of men or women in the study, thereby determining whether we had more men or women in the study (mode). We could make comparisons among variables using cross-tabulations evaluated with the chi-square statistic. Then we could determine whether a higher percentage of women as compared to men were married.

As with variables measured on a nominal scale, statistical manipulation is limited with ordinal-level variables. In addition to the mode, a median could be calculated for an ordinal scale, along with percentiles and a rank-order correlation. We could use nonparametric statistics as well. With interval-level variables, the researcher can calculate an arithmetic mean, a standard deviation, and a product moment correlation. Parametric tests, such as analysis of variance (ANOVA), are also possible. At the ratio level, all statistical tests are possible, including calculation of the geometric and harmonic mean, percentage of variation, and higher-level statistics such as regression and structured equation modeling. The student should remember that certain statistical tests, such as the t test and ANOVA, require a combination of categorical and continuous variables. For these tests, the independent variable must be categorical and the dependent variable continuous. Independent variables that are continuous can be converted into categorical variables by grouping. For example, if weight is an independent variable, it can be converted into a categorical variable by grouping participants into weight groups—those who weigh less than 100 pounds in one group and those who weigh 100 pounds or more in another.

When Stevens (1951) proposed the categorization schema and associated statistical tests, he had no idea how significant and controversial this classification would become. Yet, writing in 1959, Stevens was aware that future researchers might discover additional levels of measurement. He even proposed a logarithmic interval scale and suggested the existence of scales between the ordinal and interval levels. Some researchers, however, have applied rigid standards to the use of the schema. These investigators insist that statistics applied in any study must correspond to the appropriate level of measurement of the variables (representational view), whereas other investigators apply more flexible standards (operational or classical view; see Nunnally & Bernstein, 1994). The greatest area of controversy for behavioral researchers is the interpretation of the summated rating scales. Those who espouse the representational viewpoint insist that rating scales be evaluated using the median and nonparametric statistics. However, those in the operational and classical camps note that under certain circumstances, interval-level scales may be created from ordinal scales. One example, provided by Nunnally and Bernstein (1994), is test scores. Individual items (for example, multiple-choice or true/false) on a test are considered ordinal-level variables. However, summing the items produces an interval-level scale to which one can apply an arithmetic mean and the associated statistical tests. These statistical tests include mean comparisons (t and F tests), multiple regression, and other parametric tests. The same type of transformation is possible with summated rating scales. Individual items with response options such as *strongly disagree* to *strongly agree* are considered ordinal scales. However, summing the responses provides an interval-level variable. Nunnally and Bernstein (1994), along with others (Pedhazur & Schmelkin, 1991), note that little damage is done by the application of the higher-level statistics to the analysis of data using summated rating scales. The proof, they say, is in the results. If the literature is a reflection of health behavior researchers' beliefs in this area, most researchers are in the classical camp. A review of studies shows that it is a common practice for researchers to apply parametric statistics to the study of variables that are measured with ordinal scales, including summated rating scales.

Major Concepts of Measurement: Reliability and Validity

Reliability

The two fundamental concepts of measurement are reliability and validity. *Reliability* refers to consistency: that is, does the instrument produce scores that are internally consistent or stable across time? We do not consider a scale reliable if it indicates that a person weighs 145 pounds at one moment and 162 pounds ten minutes later (given, of course, no obvious change such as the addition of winter clothing for a trek to Kathmandu). Likewise, a thermometer is expected to provide consistent readings, as are many other instruments we use in our daily lives.

In this book we will address reliability as related to instruments designed to measure health behaviors and factors associated with health behaviors. As we will learn, several different ways to assess reliability are available. The selection of reliability procedures depends on a number of factors, including the attribute being measured, the type of instrument, the investigator's skill and available time, the availability of research participants, and data collection time and efforts. We will learn about three major procedures to assess reliability: equivalence, stability, and internal consistency.

Validity

Validity refers to the legitimacy of the scores as a measure of the intended attribute. That is, does the instrument measure what it is intended to measure? We know a thermometer measures heat, but we would not expect degrees on a thermometer to give us an indication of a person's level of self-esteem. However, measures that collect self-reports of behaviors, attitudes, and psychosocial states are not as easy to assess. Researchers encounter more difficulty in determining whether or not these measures are valid. A variety of factors—including conceptual factors, respondent factors, item factors, and methods of administration—might lead to measurement errors that would influence validity. The latest set of standards for education and psychological testing (American Educational Research Association, American Psychological Association, and National Council on Measurement in Education, 1999) lists five sources of validity evidence. These are test content, response processes, relations to other variables, internal structure, and consequences of testing. We will discuss these sources in later chapters.

Summary

Health educators and behavioral scientists holding a variety of health and research positions often need to understand measurement and to use measurement techniques. As we have learned in this chapter, measurement has a long history, dating back to ancient times. However, the measurement theories and techniques we draw on today were developed and refined primarily in the twentieth century. The work of S. S. Stevens has had a powerful impact on the conceptualization of measurement among psychologists and behavioral scientists. In particular, his definitions of measurement and categorization of variables are used extensively in instrument development and testing. In later chapters we will become familiar with the work of other giants in the field and their contributions to reliability and validity assessment.

CHAPTER TWO

TYPES OF MEASURES

LEARNING OBJECTIVES

At the end of this chapter, the student should be able to

1. List four primary methods of measuring health behaviors.
2. Compare and contrast six types of self-report measures.
3. Describe five types of rating scales.
4. Describe three uses for the observation method in health behavior research.
5. List four types of biobehavioral measures.
6. Describe two health behaviors that can be measured with electronic monitoring devices.

At the beginning of Chapter One, we briefly described a variety of roles occupied by graduates of schools of public health. You will note that the graduates were involved in several projects addressing various health issues that require the collection of data. To make decisions about data collection, the graduates must first decide on the variables to assess; then they must decide how to measure them. The purpose of this chapter is to acquaint the student with the kinds of measures available for assessing health behaviors and factors associated with health behaviors. We can classify the types of instruments broadly as self-report, observations, biobehavioral measures, and electronic monitors. The following discussion is not intended to be a detailed presentation of all aspects—both positive and negative—of these measuring devices. However, this presentation will constitute the groundwork for understanding information on the development and evaluation of measuring instruments presented in later chapters.

Self-Report

The most common types of measures used to collect data about health and health behaviors are instruments in which the participant provides a direct report of knowledge, attitudes, intentions, perceptions, or behaviors. These self-report measures include interviews, questionnaires, journals, diaries, scales and indexes; these are described in the following sections.

Interviews

Broadly defined, an interview is a special situation in which a participant is asked a question or a series of questions about a phenomenon by an individual trained in interviewing techniques. Interviews can range from relatively unstructured events to highly structured ones. Using an unstructured format, the interviewer asks one or more broad, open-ended questions about a phenomenon, to which the respondent is expected to provide detailed responses. For example, the interviewer might say, "Tell me how you stay healthy." The interviewer then guides the respondent through an in-depth discussion of the phenomenon by using probing, reflecting, and reinforcing comments. Interviewers generally use the unstructured interview approach in exploratory and qualitative research. In these situations, the researcher approaches the interview without predetermined ideas about the phenomenon. An unstructured interview is an attempt to determine what the phenomenon means to the participant in the study, rather than an attempt to validate what is already known. During the interview, the interviewer takes notes and may use a tape recorder to record the entire discussion. Later, the researcher transcribes the audiotapes and analyzes the transcripts employing a variety of techniques grounded in qualitative research methodology.

In contrast to the unstructured interview format, a highly structured interview is one in which the interviewer reads items verbatim from an interview script and records the respondent's answers. In this type of interview, interviewers generally rely on closed-ended items, in which the respondent is asked to choose from a list of response options. They ask few if any open-ended questions. If they do include open-ended questions, the requested response is generally short (for example, Question: *What is your favorite type of exercise?* Response: *Running*). In health behavioral studies, researchers commonly collect data using the structured-interview format.

A semistructured interview is one that combines elements of both unstructured and highly structured interviews. Researchers include both open-ended and closed-ended questions. Thus, in one approach, an interviewer might ask a respondent to answer a series of closed-ended items and then to clarify selected responses by providing more detail. In another approach, an interviewer might begin the discussion by asking an open-ended question and then probe for more specific details using closed-ended questions. Researchers use the semistructured interview when they want to explore a range of opinions, perceptions, and attitudes about a specific topic. Although the research can be exploratory, the researcher is usually interested in a specific aspect of the phenomenon.

Focus group scripts are excellent examples of the semistructured interview. Researchers convene focus groups for a variety of reasons, including generating items for questionnaires, gathering feasibility data during the pilot phase of a study, or obtaining perspectives on the results of a study during the interpretation phase. The purpose of the focus group is fairly specific and the researchers generally have a good understanding of the type of information they want to collect. However, they lack a full appreciation of the range of opinions and ideas that people hold about the topic.

Questionnaires

Questionnaire is a general term used to describe instruments that consist of items answered directly by the respondent. The usual format for the questionnaire is paper-and-pencil, and the items on the questionnaire are predominantly closed-ended questions. Recent advances in computer technology now allow respondents to complete questionnaires using a computer. A survey is a special type of questionnaire designed to address specific research questions. Most surveys consist primarily of closed-ended items. In practice, we often use the terms *questionnaire* and *survey* interchangeably. Sometimes the manner of administration of the questionnaire determines

---

Open- and Closed-Ended Questions

Responses to closed-ended questions (also called forced-choice responses) are predetermined, so that the respondent selects the best answer for him or her from a list of two or more answer choices. Open-ended questions allow respondents to compose their own responses. Responses to closed-ended questions are easier to code for statistical analysis, but the responses lack detail. Open-ended questions generate variability in responses, more detail, and more precise responses. However, analysis of data is more complex.

the term used to refer to it. For example, we refer to a questionnaire administered in a face-to-face meeting by a trained interviewer as a structured interview. We generally call a questionnaire administered over the telephone by a trained interviewer a telephone survey, and one mailed to a respondent's home a mail survey.

A questionnaire or survey can contain a single type of item or a variety of types. Examples of types of items that a questionnaire or survey might include follow.

A simple item is one in which the respondent chooses between two options, such as *yes/no, male/female,* and *married/not married.* For example:

What is your sex?

_____ Male

_____ Female

Another simple type of item requires a short written response.

What is your age? _____

How many fruits did you eat yesterday? _____

Another example of a simple item is one in which participants rate their attitudes, their opinions, or their health using a response scale. Response scales can consist of two options (these are called dichotomous) or more.

Medicare should pay for prescription medications for all Americans over 65 years of age.

_____ Agree   _____ Disagree

How would you rate your health?

_____ Excellent

_____ Good

_____ Average

_____ Poor

_____ Very poor

Researchers employ multiple-choice and true/false items primarily to assess knowledge. Examples are

HIV is caused by a bacterium.

_____ True _____ False

The variable *marital status* is usually measured on what type of scale?

A. Nominal

B. Ordinal

C. Interval

D. Ratio

Checklists, such as the following, are often used to obtain information on medical histories.

Which of the following health conditions have you ever had? (Check ✓ all that apply.)

_____ Anemia

_____ Asthma

_____ Diabetes

_____ Ear infection

_____ Heart disease

_____ High blood pressure

_____ Seizures

_____ Sinus infection

A questionnaire can also include other types of items, such as those that require the ranking of items or those that require short responses. The type of item, the length of the questionnaire, and the questionnaire format depend on a variety of factors, including the expertise of the researcher, the type of respondent (including age and education), and the mode of delivery (telephone, mail, face-to-face, or computer assessment). (Chapter Seven discusses item development.)

Journals and Diaries

Journals and diaries are used to collect data about events, feelings, emotions, and beliefs. Journaling is an activity in which a respondent writes detailed notes about thoughts and experiences. When used in health behavior research, journaling is related to a health event, perhaps one's experiences related to the diagnosis and treatment of breast cancer. The information obtained from a journal is treated much like data collected through unstructured interviews. Researchers read the journal entries and categorize feelings, attitudes, behaviors, and events according to general themes. Journaling tends to generate a large amount of information that requires considerable time to process, code, and analyze. Because of these drawbacks, journaling is not a common method of measuring health-related variables.

A diary is similar to a journal in that the researcher asks the respondent to record events and emotional or cognitive elements of those events. The research diary, however, tends to be more structured than the journal. Researchers might ask participants to record what they eat during a twenty-four-hour period as a means of measuring food or nutrient intake. Researchers might also ask respondents to use a calendar to record seizures, side effects of medications, symptoms associated with illness or treatments, headaches, arrhythmias, exercise, or physical activity.

Response Scales

The response scale is one of the more common approaches for collecting data on opinions, perceptions, and attitudes. A response scale asks respondents to select, on a scale, a point that most closely represents their position from low to high or from negative to positive. The first use of a response scale has been attributed to Hipparchus, who is noted to have used a six-point scale in 150 B.C. to assess the brightness of stars (Lodge, 1981). Response scales represent graduated increments of agreement, frequency, or evaluation (Spector, 1992). Using a scale that assesses agreement, respondents indicate how much they agree with a particular statement: for frequency, respondents indicate how often they perform a particular behavior; for the evaluative scale, respondents rate items according to how positive or negative they feel about them.

FIGURE 2.1. RESPONSE FORMAT FROM A WORKSHEET COMPLETED BY A FIRST-GRADE STUDENT.

I liked this story

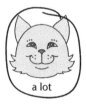

a lot   some   a little   not much

I liked the way I worked today

  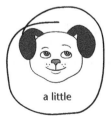

a lot   some   a little   not much

FIGURE 2.2. WONG-BAKER FACES PAIN RATING SCALE.

Faces Pain Rating Scale

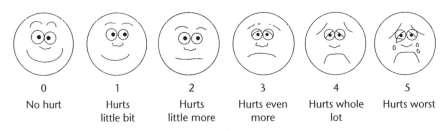

0	1	2	3	4	5
No hurt	Hurts little bit	Hurts little more	Hurts even more	Hurts whole lot	Hurts worst

Source: Wong, D. L., M. Hockenberry-Eaton, D. Wilson, M. L. Winkelstein, and P. Schwartz, *Wong's Essentials of Pediatric Nursing,* 6th ed., St. Louis, 2001, p. 1301. Copyrighted by Mosby, Inc. Reprinted by permission.

Response scales come in a variety of formats, some of which are depicted in Figures 2.1 and 2.2 and Exhibit 2.1. Depending on the type of response scale, the respondent might circle a number, letter, word, or figure; insert a check mark (✓) or X, or draw a line to mark a respondent's position on a continuum.

Scaling Methods

Scaling is a process whereby researchers use a set of items to measure behaviors, attitudes, or feelings. The most common reason for scaling is to obtain a single score that represents a person's overall attitude, belief, or behavior about a given situation or object (Trochim, 2001). Several forms of scaling exist; there are specific rules for developing and using each scale. In Chapter Seven, we present procedures for the development of scales. Here, we describe five types: the visual analog scale (VAS), the Thurstone scale, the Likert scale, the Guttman scale, and the semantic differential rating scale (SD). The VAS and the Likert scales are the most commonly used scales in health behavior research, followed by the SD. Although the Thurstone and Guttman scales are presented here, they are rarely used in health behavior research. However, because these scales are frequently cited, students should be familiar with them and appreciate the reasons they are rarely selected as methods for data collection.

Visual Analog Scale. The visual analog scale is a type of graphic rating scale. The concept underlying the VAS dates back to Freyd, who in 1923 described a similar procedure for use in assessing personality traits (Freyd, 1923). During the past thirty years, the VAS has gained popularity in health behavior research and evaluation

EXHIBIT 2.1. EXAMPLES OF RESPONSE FORMATS.

Place an X on the line that most closely reflects the extent to which you agree or disagree with each statement.

The instructor seemed knowledgeable about the subject matter.

Agree _____ _____ _____ _____ Disagree

Circle the word that most closely reflects the extent to which you agree or disagree with each statement.

The instructor seemed knowledgeable about the subject matter.

Strongly agree   Agree   Disagree   Strongly disagree

Circle the number that corresponds most closely to the extent of your agreement with each statement.

The instructor seemed knowledgeable about the subject matter.

Strongly agree   Agree   Disagree   Strongly disagree
   1   2   3   4

Circle the number that corresponds most closely to the extent of your agreement with each statement.

1 = Strongly disagree   10 = Strongly agree

The instructor seemed knowledgeable about the subject matter.

 1   2   3   4   5   6   7   8   9   10

because of its simplicity. Researchers have used the VAS to measure a variety of health phenomena, including pain, nausea, fatigue, and anxiety.

The most basic type of VAS consists of a straight horizontal or vertical line, 100 mm long. At each end, the scale developer places a perpendicular line, to clearly mark the starting and ending points of the line. Terms depicting extreme positions anchor the end points. For example, a VAS to measure pain might have anchor phrases of *no pain* and *pain as bad as it could be*. A VAS to measure anxiety could have the anchor phrases *not nervous at all* and *the most nervous I have ever been* (Cline, Herman, et al., 1992). The respondent marks the point on the line that corresponds most closely to his or her position on the phenomenon being assessed at that moment. Each respondent's numeric score is calculated by measuring the distance from one end of the line to the respondent's mark on the line. The length of this distance is considered to be the respondent's score.

The 100 mm line has special significance because it allows the researcher to measure the amount of the phenomenon on a continuous scale from 0 (none of the phenomenon) to 100 (maximum amount). Traditional response scales requiring a selection

FIGURE 2.3. GENERAL FORM OF A VISUAL ANALOG SCALE.

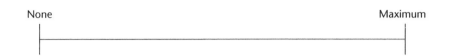

of one of several responses (for example, *agree* or *disagree*) fall in the category of ordinal scales. Although it is possible to rank scores from low to high, one cannot assume that people with the same score have exactly the same amount of the attribute or that there is an equal amount of the attribute between each pair of points on the scale. The VAS more closely approximates the continuous scale (Price, McGrath, et al., 1983).

A number of variants of the simple form of the VAS exist (Paul-Dauphin, Guillemin, et al., 1999). In addition to the simple line with anchors, a VAS might include a perpendicular line at the midpoint or perpendicular lines at equal intervals along the line (graduated VAS). These gradations might include numbers (10, 20, 30, and so on) or verbal descriptors (*not at all, a little, moderately, a lot*) or both. Another type of VAS eliminates the line and includes only numbers, with verbal anchors at the ends. To make the task appealing to respondents, some researchers use familiar devices such as ladders or thermometers to depict the attribute and the end points.

Thurstone Scale. In the 1920s, L. L. Thurstone (Thurstone & Chave, 1929) made a major breakthrough in the measurement of attitudes. Thurstone believed that asking people about their preferences would be more interesting and perhaps more relevant for the study of psychology than sensory-stimuli testing (for example, just noticeable differences in weight). His work led to the development of three scaling methods: equal-appearing intervals, paired comparisons, and successive intervals. In each approach, respondents are asked to select from a set of items those that they endorse. Each item has a preassigned weight, and researchers add the preassigned weights for the items that are endorsed to obtain a total score. The three approaches differ in the ways in which the weights are determined for the items. Here we will describe the methods for determining the weights for the equal-appearing interval approach to attitude measurement.

This process begins with the development of a large set of items (about 100) related to the attitude to be assessed. Judges who are experts in the area are asked to sort the items into eleven piles from lowest to highest according to the strength or desirability of the attitude. After the judges are satisfied with their rankings, the researcher evaluates each item individually. The values of the ranks given to the items by the judges are placed in order from high to low. The middle (median) rank value is selected as the weight for each item. The final step is to select a representative set of items from the total set. This process is carried out by rank-ordering the items according to their median weights and selecting items that represent the full range of scores, with equal intervals between successive items. An example will help clarify the process.

A researcher who plans to develop a Thurstone scale to assess attitudes toward people with epilepsy begins by writing items that express positive, negative, and neutral attitudes about people with epilepsy. These items might include such statements as, "People with epilepsy should not drive," and, "People with epilepsy can do anything anyone else can do." After writing and editing 100 items, the researcher gives the items to experts on epilepsy and asks them to sort the items into eleven piles from most negative to most positive attitudes. To make the task easier, the researcher puts each item on a separate card. After the judges are satisfied with the rankings they have assigned to all the items, the researcher evaluates items individually. Suppose that the rank values of the judges for the item "People with epilepsy can do anything they want" are as follows: 6, 6, 7, 7, 8, 8, 8, 9, 9, 9. The median value is 8, and this value is selected as the weight for the item. To select the final set of items for this scale, the items are put in order (piles) by their median values, and ten items are selected (Exhibit 2.2). These ten items have values ranging from 1 to 10, with one point between successive items. When using the scale, a person who agrees with the statement "People with epilepsy can do anything anyone else can do" will receive a score of 8; a person who agrees with the statement "People with epilepsy should not drive" will receive a score of 3. Total scores are found by adding together the rank value of each item to which the respondent agrees. On this scale, higher scores correspond to more positive attitudes toward people with epilepsy.

EXHIBIT 2.2. EXAMPLE OF A THURSTONE SCALE, USING HYPOTHETICAL ITEMS AND WEIGHTS FOR AN EPILEPSY ATTITUDE SCALE.

Item (weight)	Agree	Disagree
1. People with epilepsy can do anything they want. (8)	1	2
2. People with epilepsy should not drive. (3)	1	2
3. People with epilepsy should not get married. (4)	1	2
4. People with epilepsy should not be around heavy machinery. (6)	1	2
5. People with epilepsy are mentally ill. (1)	1	2
6. People with epilepsy should not have children. (2)	1	2
7. People with epilepsy can hold important positions. (9)	1	2
8. People with epilepsy cannot hold a job. (5)	1	2
9. People with epilepsy should be treated like anyone else. (10)	1	2
10. People with epilepsy make a valuable contribution to society. (7)	1	2

Note: Numbers in parentheses correspond to the rank value of the item.

Likert Scale. Rensis Likert (Likert, 1932), among others, liked Thurstone's idea of measuring preferences but believed that the method of weighting items was time-consuming and cumbersome. For his dissertation, Likert developed a simple approach to constructing attitudinal scales. The Likert scale, also called a summated rating scale, is now the most widely used scale for measuring behaviors, attitudes, and feelings. The Likert scale builds on the concept of the one-item response scale. Rather than using one item to measure the totality of an attribute, the scale uses several items to assess an attribute. Respondents rate each item individually, and the responses are added to obtain a total score.

The Rosenberg Self-Esteem Scale (Rosenberg, 1965, 1989) is a good example of a Likert scale. Rosenberg developed this scale in 1965 to measure self-esteem among adolescents and adults (Table 2.1). The participant is first asked to respond to each item by circling the number that best represents his or her level of agreement. To obtain a total score on the Rosenberg Self-Esteem Scale, researchers add the responses to each item. Note that items numbered 3, 5, 8, 9, and 10 are negatively worded. That is, strong agreement with these items indicates a low level of self-esteem. By contrast, items numbered 1, 2, 4, 6, and 7 are positively worded, so that strong agreement with them is consistent with a high level of self-esteem. To compute a total score for the scale, the negatively worded items must first be reverse-scored. To reverse-score items, researchers code responses to the items in an order opposite to their numerical order. For example, with the Rosenberg Self-Esteem Scale, a response of 1 to a negatively worded item is coded 4; a response of 2 is coded 3; a response of 3 is coded

---

Negatively Worded Items

Negatively worded items on a scale are those items to which strong agreement would indicate low levels of the concept. A negatively worded item on a happiness scale might be "I do not feel cheerful most of the time." A high level of agreement with this item would indicate a low level of happiness. Another negatively worded item might be "I feel sad," because a high level of agreement with this item also would indicate a low level of happiness. Note that the first item, "I do not feel cheerful most of the time," includes the word *not,* but the second item, "I feel sad," does not. The term *negatively worded item* refers not to the grammatical negativity of the statement, but to the way the response to the item corresponds to the concept. If depression were the concept under consideration, both of these items would be considered positively worded, and the item "I feel happy" would be considered a negatively worded item.

TABLE 2.1. THE ROSENBERG SELF-ESTEEM SCALE.

Below is a list of statements dealing with your general feelings about yourself. If you strongly agree, circle SA. If you agree, circle A. If you disagree, circle D. If you strongly disagree, circle SD.

	1. Strongly Agree	2. Agree	3. Disagree	4. Strongly Disagree
1. I feel that I'm a person of worth, at least on an equal plane with others.	SA	A	D	SD
2. I feel that I have a number of good qualities.	SA	A	D	SD
3. All in all, I am inclined to feel that I am a failure.[a]	SA	A	D	SD
4. I am able to do things as well as most other people.	SA	A	D	SD
5. I feel I do not have much to be proud of.[a]	SA	A	D	SD
6. I take a positive attitude toward myself.	SA	A	D	SD
7. On the whole, I am satisfied with myself.	SA	A	D	SD
8. I wish I could have more respect for myself.[a]	SA	A	D	SD
9. I certainly feel useless at times.[a]	SA	A	D	SD
10. At times I think I am no good at all.[a]	SA	A	D	SD

[a] Reverse-scored items

Source: Rosenberg, M. (1989). *Society and the Adolescent Self-Image.* Revised edition. Middletown, Conn.: Wesleyan University Press. Used by permission.

2; and a response of 4 is coded 1. By reverse-scoring the negatively worded items, we reverse the scale so that higher scores for each item correspond to a more positive response for that item. Once the negatively worded items are reverse-scored, we can compute a total score. To compute a total score, the score for each item is summed. For the Rosenberg Self-Esteem Scale, total possible scores range from 10 to 40, and the higher scores correspond to higher levels of self-esteem.

Guttman Scale. Louis Guttman (1944) developed his scaling approach in the 1940s. The Guttman scale is unique in that the items are constructed in such a way that an affirmative response to one item in a set suggests affirmative responses to previous (or later) items in that set. A person's total score on the scale is obtained by counting the number of items answered in the affirmative.

For example, here is a set of items that we could include in a physical activity questionnaire.

Please answer the following items about your current ability to run. Circle *Yes* or *No* for each item.

1.	I can run 20 feet.	Yes	No
2.	I can run 1 block.	Yes	No
3.	I can run 1 mile.	Yes	No
4.	I can run 5 miles.	Yes	No
5.	I can run 10 miles.	Yes	No
6.	I can run a marathon (26.2 miles).	Yes	No

In this set of items, we expect that a person who reports that he or she can run a marathon would also agree with items 1 through 5: "I can run 20 feet," "I can run 1 block," "I can run 1 mile," "I can run 5 miles," and "I can run 10 miles." People who state that they can run 26.2 miles are unlikely to say that they cannot run 5 miles.

We find total scores on cumulative scales by summing affirmative responses. In this case, a person who can run a maximum of 20 feet would receive a score of 1, whereas a person who can run a marathon would likely respond *yes* to all six items and receive a score of 6. Guttman scaling works well with functional abilities, such as discrete types of physical activity or developmental milestones in children. However, constructing a set of items to measure attitudes or beliefs that can be arranged in an ascending (or descending) order of agreement is more difficult.

Semantic Differential Rating Scale. Osgood developed the semantic differential scale to assess the meanings of concepts (Osgood, 1952). SD scales generally assess meaning along three dimensions: evaluation, potency, and activity. To assess these dimensions, respondents rate a selected concept using a set of bipolar adjectives. The adjectives are selected to represent the three dimensions. Thus, evaluation might be represented by *bad/good, nice/awful,* and *fair/unfair;* potency by *small/large, weak/strong,* and *hard/soft;* and activity by *active/passive, slow/fast,* and *sharp/dull.*
Here is an example of an SD:

Instructions: Below are two concepts, "mother" and "people over 65 years of age." Beneath each concept is a list of paired adjectives. Each pair of adjectives represents opposite views. To show how you feel about each of the concepts "mother" and "people over 65 years of age," place an X on one of the lines between each adjective pair. The closer you put the X to an adjective in the pair, the more you agree with that adjective and the less you agree with its opposite. Place an X on the middle line if you are neutral or unsure of your feelings.

Mother

Good _____ _____ _____ _____ _____ _____ _____ Bad

Hard _____ _____ _____ _____ _____ _____ _____ Soft

Active _____ _____ _____ _____ _____ _____ ____ Passive

People over 65 years of age

Nice _____ _____ _____ _____ _____ _____ _____ Awful

Weak _____ _____ _____ _____ _____ _____ ____ Strong

Fast _____ _____ _____ _____ _____ _____ _____ Slow

Typically, seven lines are placed between each pair of adjectives in an SD. For scoring purposes, we code the lines from 1 to 7. The numeric value given corresponds to the number assigned to that line. Thus, a mark at the far left would be coded as 1 and one at the far right as 7. Notice that some positive adjectives are on the right and some are on the left. Before summing, researchers must reverse-score some items so that all the items are scored in the same direction. That is, the total score should reflect the extent to which the respondent has a positive or negative view of the concept. Occasionally, researchers have combined the SD format with the VAS format so that a straight, solid 100 mm line connects the bipolar adjectives. In these cases, they determine the respondent's score by measuring the distance from one end of the line to the respondent's mark. For consistency, the researcher must decide whether to measure always from the more positive or always from the more negative adjective.

Indexes

An index, like a scale, consists of a set of items (Bollen & Lennox, 1991). There are two major differences between an index and a scale. The first is that the response options for items composing an index can vary, whereas for a scale, the response options are either the same (for example, an *agree/disagree* response scale) or similar (for example, the rating of bipolar adjectives on the SD). Exhibit 2.3 shows a set of items that make up an index of socioeconomic status. Notice that unlike scales, in which each item is generally rated using the same response options, this index has, for each of the items in it, a different set of response options. Another type of index might consist of a checklist of events or situations and respondents might check those that apply to them. For example, an index of life stress might include a list of stressful events such as death in the family, divorce, marriage, birth, new job, or job loss. A second difference between an index and a scale is the relationships among the items. We will learn in Chapter Ten that a desired aspect of scales is that the items composing a scale be positively correlated with one another. In contrast, items composing an index might be positively correlated with each other, but they also might show no correlation with other items on the index (Bollen & Lennox, 1991). An index created to measure complexity of medication regimens might include the dose and frequency of a medication as well as actions required to take the medication (for example, injection or breaking a pill in half). The number of doses required per day may have no correlation with the number or type of actions required to take the medication. Total scores on an index are found most often by summing responses to individual items. However, an investigator might weight items differently depending on the overall contribution of each item to the construct being measured.

EXHIBIT 2.3. EXAMPLES OF ITEMS FOR AN INDEX OF SOCIOECONOMIC STATUS.

1. What is your highest level of education?

    1. _____ Eleventh grade or less
    2. _____ High school graduate
    3. _____ Some college or technical school
    4. _____ Graduated from technical school
    5. _____ Graduated from college
    6. _____ Postgraduate study
    7. _____ Graduate degree

2. What best describes your yearly household income?

    1. _____ Less than $20,000
    2. _____ $20,000–$49,999
    3. _____ $50,000–$74,999
    4. _____ $75,000–$99,999
    5. _____ $100,000 or more

3. What type of work do you do? _____

4. Do you own a home?

    1. _____ Yes (Go to Question 5)
    2. _____ No (Stop)

5. If yes, what is the current market value of your home?

    1. _____ Less than $100,000
    2. _____ $100,000–$149,999
    3. _____ $150,000–$199,999
    4. _____ $200,000–$299,999
    5. _____ $300,000–$499,999
    6. _____ $500,000 or more

Observations

Whereas rating scales are the most common method of collecting data on health behaviors and associated factors, observations are among the least used strategies for collecting health behavior data. Although observations can provide extensive information, which in some cases is more accurate than that from self-report, they are time-consuming and expensive. In addition, when relying on observations, investigators must establish procedures to assess reliability each time, thus increasing the time and expense for the collection of data. Despite these drawbacks, researchers still use observations to collect interesting data, particularly in areas of health behavior where self-report is limited. Behavioral intervention studies to assess fidelity to interventions also benefit from the observation approach.

When properly performed, a systematic observation includes careful identification of the behaviors to observe, definitions of the behaviors to evaluate, examples of what constitutes each behavior and what does not, development of a protocol for the observation, and training of the observers. Most important, observers follow specific protocols to identify and classify behaviors of interest to researchers. Thus, the observation process is more rigorous than simply viewing an event or situation.

The types of behaviors that researchers have observed systematically are quite varied and include conversations, interactions, body movements, facial expressions, and reactions. These researchers have relied on observations to code emotions, such as aggression, anger, empathy, and comfort; verbal statements, including quality or tone; and distance between participants (personal space). For the selected behavior, observers identify the presence or absence of the behavior, its frequency, and/or its intensity. Generally, observers use response scales (occurrence, frequency, intensity) or checklists to record their observations. Before data collection, the researcher trains observers to observe and code the behavior.

Biobehavioral Measures

Biobehavioral measures are a variety of physical measures that are used to assess health behavior outcomes. These include physiological measures, such as heart rate and blood pressure, and anthropometric measures, such as height and weight. A researcher who is interested in evaluating an intervention to promote adherence to hypertension medication might measure medication blood levels to evaluate the success of the intervention. A researcher who is conducting a program to compare strength training to endurance training might measure fitness using a measure of oxygen consumption. Blood tests such as those for cholesterol, blood sugar, HIV, strep throat, chlamydia, and hemoglobin might all be used to assess some aspect of health behavior outcome for behavioral studies.

Biobehavioral measures are generally considered to be more objective measures of health status than are self-report measures. For example, a person may be likely to respond *no* on a questionnaire about having a sexually transmitted disease but may show evidence of gonorrhea with urine testing. Likewise, a respondent may say he or she always takes his or her medications, but a blood test may show low levels of the drug. Because biobehavioral measures are seen as more objective measures in some cases, researchers are encouraged to include them in their studies when possible.

Electronic Measures

Advances in technology have led to the development of a number of electronic measures for a variety of health behaviors. Investigators use many of these measures to augment self-reports of behaviors that are difficult or impossible to observe. One example is a pedometer, usually worn over one hip to measure physical activity. Movement of the hip activates a pendulum within the device, and movement of the pendulum in turn activates a gear linked to a digital display that shows number of "footsteps" (Bassey, Dallosso, et al., 1987). When the average length of a "footstep" is entered, the device converts steps into miles. Although the pedometer can provide an estimate of distance traveled, precise measurement of physical activity and energy expenditure is not possible using this instrument (Kashiwazaki, Inaoka, et al., 1986; Bassey, Dallosso, et al., 1987). The reason is that steps generally vary in length, and energy expenditure varies depending on the intensity of the movement.

Another device, used to measure medication use, is the electronic event monitor (AARDEX, Ltd., 2005). This device consists of a cap that fits on standard medication bottles. Within the cap is a small computer chip with a counter to record each time the cap is removed. The chip is also programmed with date and time information, and thus can record the date and time of every cap removal. When the cap is removed, presumably when the person takes his or her medications, the computer chip records the date and time of removal. The chip cannot record the number of pills taken out or the actual ingestion of the medication, but it can provide a record from which the researcher can determine whether the person is remembering to open the bottle at times corresponding to a medication schedule. The information contained in the cap can be transferred to a computer, and using software that interfaces with the device, researchers can obtain information on the number of times the cap is removed each day, the time of each removal, the number of times it was removed according to the prescribed schedule, and the percentage of times the bottle was opened according to schedule. Researchers have used electronic event monitors in a number of research studies, and they have found these to be reliable and valid measures of adherence (Cramer, Mattson, et al., 1989; Favre, Delacretaz, et al., 1997).

Summary

As can be seen from the discussion in this chapter, health educators and behavioral scientists have a variety of instruments at their disposal. Each type of instrument has strengths and weaknesses, and each must be evaluated individually to determine its usefulness for any particular project or study. Self-report measures are the most common type of instrument used in behavior research and program evaluation. Of the self-report measures, single-item questions and summated rating scales are the most frequently used approaches to data collection. Thus, health researchers have spent considerable time and effort in developing these instruments and testing their reliability and validity. Because of the importance of self-report measures in health studies, we will focus on them in the following chapters.

CHAPTER THREE

MEASUREMENT ERROR

LEARNING OBJECTIVES

At the end of this chapter, the student should be able to

1. Define measurement error.
2. Define and give examples of random measurement error.
3. Define and give examples of systematic measurement error.
4. Compare and contrast random and systematic error.
5. List five respondent factors associated with measurement error.
6. Identify and describe five types of response sets.
7. Describe three ways to minimize measurement error due to respondent factors.
8. List five instrument factors associated with measurement error.
9. Describe three ways to minimize measurement error due to instrument factors.
10. List three situational factors associated with measurement error.
11. Describe two ways to minimize measurement error due to situational factors.

In Chapter One we mentioned that error in the course of measurement is inevitable. The pervasiveness of measurement error is captured by the adage "Measure twice, cut once." And the quandary faced when errors do occur is reflected in Brennan's axiom (2001, p. 2): "A person with one watch knows the time of day. A person with two watches is never quite sure what time it is." Because measurement error is ubiquitous by nature, people learn to tolerate some degree of error in daily life. As adults, most of us are willing to accept a fluctuation of 1 to 2 pounds in our body weight if it is measured each day. We often attribute these weight fluctuations to changes in hydration or the consumption of more or less food in a given day. For a five-day-old infant, a gain or loss of 1 pound over a twenty-four-hour period has an entirely different meaning. Either this percentage of body weight change is due to a gross measurement error or it reflects a serious medical condition. In either case, the cause of the weight change must immediately be investigated. In situations in which large or unexpected changes occur and are due to faulty measurement, we are less tolerant of error and seek both to determine the cause and to prevent a repetition of the error. In health research and evaluation, serious measurement errors can yield flawed data and false conclusions. For health professionals, it is important to understand the sources of measurement error and learn strategies for minimizing or eliminating it when we are assessing health-related concepts.

We begin this chapter by defining measurement error in the context of psychometric theory. We then discuss random and systematic errors, which are the two major classes of errors. Random and systematic errors can be attributed to three broad factors: respondents, instruments, and situations. Each of these factors is discussed, along with strategies that investigators can use to reduce or prevent errors.

Definition

We have introduced the concepts of reliability and validity. The term *reliability* refers to the consistency of scores obtained from a measure, and the term *validity* refers to the legitimacy of the scores as a measure of the chosen attribute. Although we expect that any measure we use will be appropriate for the population from which we plan to gather data and will yield perfectly accurate scores each time we use it, this is never the case. No measure ever produces perfectly reliable or valid scores. We refer to the extent to which a measure deviates from the ideal level of reliability and validity as *measurement error.*

Definition of the Term Test

In the context of measurement, *test* is a general term that refers to a number of different types of measures, including measures of knowledge, attitudes, skills, or behaviors. In this book, we use the term to refer primarily to knowledge tests and to scales that measure attitudes, behaviors, and other health concepts.

Classification of Measurement Error

Random Error

The two basic types of measurement error are *random* and *systematic*. Random error is due to chance factors that influence the measurement of a variable. As its name implies, random error is an unsystematic error. It does not affect the attribute being measured in the same way each time a measurement is taken. For example, a student taking an exam might misread items and circle wrong answers due to inattention, fatigue, or distraction and consequently obtain a score that suggests a lower level of knowledge about the subject matter than the student actually possesses. On the next exam, the student might guess on several questions and select the correct answers without actually knowing the information, thereby achieving a score that suggests a higher level of knowledge than he or she has. In both cases, random error has occurred—once to the detriment of the student and once in the student's favor. However, in each case, random events occurred that resulted in errors of measurement.

Viswanathan (2005) classifies random error as *generic* or *idiosyncratic*. Generic random errors affect a large proportion of the respondents, whereas idiosyncratic errors affect a small proportion of respondents. Survey items that are ambiguous, instructions that are hard to follow, and testing situations that are uncomfortable (for example, heat or noise) are likely to elicit response errors among a broad group of respondents and thus are classified as generic random error. Individual characteristics such as fatigue, hunger, and distraction are more likely to affect a small group of respondents within the sample.

Random error is important to understand because it affects the reliability of a measure. A perfectly reliable instrument is one in which the same score is obtained on repeated measurements of an attribute, provided there is no change in the attribute. Thus, if we measured the length of a table, we would expect to obtain the same result each time we measured it. If the table is 32 inches long, it should measure 32 inches each time. However, because measurement is fallible, we are likely to obtain three slightly different results if we measure the table three times. We may attribute the differences to failure to place the beginning or end of the ruler at the same point each time or to lack of precision in reading the number of inches. A person asked to record fruit and vegetable intake each day for a week may forget to record an orange one day and mistakenly list a banana another day. Researchers expect slight errors in measurement, and these small idiosyncratic errors are unlikely to affect reliability to a great extent (Viswanathan, 2005). Indeed, if we take many independent measures of an attribute, most likely the positive and negative errors will cancel each other, and the average of all the measurements will reflect the actual score a person might have obtained without error. Consider the student taking an exam. If the student inadvertently circles a wrong answer, but then guesses correctly on another item, the errors cancel each other, and the total score is a true reflection of the student's knowledge of the subject matter. In contrast, generic random error, which affects a large proportion of the respondents, may affect the reliability of the measure. Students taking an exam that has numerous typographical errors, ambiguous response choices, and an inadequate format may obtain widely different scores on two successive administrations of that test. The test would be considered an unreliable indicator of the students' knowledge of the subject matter.

Systematic Error

Systematic error is due to factors that systematically increase or decrease true scores of an attribute. For example, a scale to measure weight that is calibrated incorrectly might consistently add 2 pounds to each person's weight. In this case, the scale would provide a consistent measure of weight, but that measure would always be 2 pounds more than a respondent's actual weight. Other examples of systematic error include incorrect directions on a questionnaire that lead respondents to record their responses in the wrong place, and a scale designed to measure depression that also measures fatigue. In each case, the instrument may be reliable; investigators might obtain the same results on repeated use of the instrument. However, each time they use the instrument, they repeat the systematic error, affecting the extent to which the instrument actually measures the attribute. Thus, systematic error has its greatest effect on the validity of a measure. Systematic error causes scores to be inaccurate, and, if it is extreme, it can limit the usefulness of the measuring instrument.

Systematic error can be categorized as *additive* or *correlational* systematic error (Viswanathan, 2005). Additive systematic error was described earlier and refers to a consistent deviation from the true score in the same direction (for example, always adding 2 pounds to one's weight). Correlational systematic error occurs when measures consistently inflate or deflate scores but do so in different ways for different respondents. Some survey respondents, for example, may consistently answer more positively than they actually feel to items and others may answer more negatively. Though the individual respondents' deviations are in the same direction, the overall sample is composed of responses that are sometimes inflated and sometimes deflated.

Another type of systematic error is bias. This kind of systematic error fails to affect the entire group of respondents, but does affect one or more subgroups of respondents (Camilli & Shepard, 1994). One group may be more prone, or biased, to answer items in a certain way because of age, gender, education, or cultural background.

In the early 1900s, Alfred Binet was aware of bias in the development of items for the IQ test (Binet & Simon, 1973). He noted that certain items tended to differentiate children by economic status rather than by intelligence. Thus, he included only items found to measure consistently across the socioeconomic statuses of the children. He eliminated items that seemed to be dependent on home or school training.

Although test developers knew for many years that this type of bias existed, its presence did not gain national prominence until the 1960s and 1970s. The civil rights movement raised awareness of the possible cultural bias of standardized tests, and concern grew over those tests used to make important decisions such as college admission (Camilli & Shepard, 1994).

The content of some portions of standardized tests may favor certain groups. For example, males may find a reading section about baseball more appealing and easier to understand because they have a tendency to follow baseball more closely than females do. Analogies such as "*trot* is to *canter* as *jog* is to *run*" favor a test taker who is familiar with the movements of horses. As a result of the concerns expressed by various cultural groups in the United States, test developers have examined bias in testing more carefully, and extensive efforts are currently under way to include culturally diverse reading passages, word problems, and vocabulary items.

Measurement Error Factors

Errors in measurement arise from several sources that are broadly classified as errors due to the respondent, the instrument, or the situation. Below we describe some examples of each of these three sources of error.

Respondent Factors

In completing self-report questionnaires and interviews, respondents can make a number of errors. Possible respondent errors include

- Overreporting or underreporting agreement with items
- Overreporting or underreporting frequency of events
- Overreporting or underreporting positive or negative attitudes
- Giving partial answers
- Giving inconsistent answers
- Making recording errors, such as putting a response in the wrong place

The reasons that test takers make errors are as numerous as the possible types of errors. However, common reasons for making errors include simply misunderstanding what information was requested; maturation issues, such as fatigue and boredom; lack of interest or time; carelessness or guessing; copying; and failure to attend to instructions.

The study of how people respond to items on questionnaires has led to a greater understanding of the cognitive processes that people use to answer questions (Tourangeau & Rasinski, 1988) as well as to the identification of several patterns that people sometimes follow in responding to items. The literature often refers to these patterns as response sets or biases.

In reference to the cognitive processes that people use in answering items, the respondent assumes an attitude that may help him or her complete the task in an optimal manner or, conversely, one that may undermine the task and lead to more respondent error. Krosnick (1991) coined the term *optimizing* to refer to the situation in which people approach self-report tasks with the optimal mental attitude. People who take this approach use their mental resources to complete the questionnaire in the best way they can. They give each item full consideration and try to provide the best answer. Academic examinations offer the best example of optimizing. Here, students who are interested in doing well on a test read each item carefully, think about possible responses, and carefully record their answers. People who want to participate in clinical trials to receive treatment for a specific disorder, or who want to qualify for a particular event such as a reality show (for example, *Survivor*), might also try their best by carefully reading instructions, answering questions, and recording answers. Krosnick (1991) notes that optimizing is the ideal attitude that people may assume when responding to self-report questionnaires. Because people are trying to give the appropriate information when optimizing, this situation results in the smallest amount of respondent error.

People who are not particularly invested in completing a specific questionnaire might opt for *a satisficing rather than an optimizing approach*. Krosnick (1991) used the term *satisficing* to mean giving the answer that seems most reasonable at the time. People who take a satisficing approach pay less attention to what is asked, spend less time considering their answers, and offer a "good enough" response. This mental attitude is probably most common among students taking a quiz that will not greatly affect their course grades or among people who do not have strong feelings about an issue but are asked to complete a survey about it. Because people fail to give as much care to responding to items, the likelihood of making an error—for example, failure to follow directions, recording errors, and overreporting or underreporting attitudes—is greater for this group than for people with an optimizing attitude.

On the far end of the continuum are people who apply a negative attitude in responding to items (Silverman, 1977). A person might display a negative attitude if that person felt coerced into completing a survey, then discovered survey bias toward a view opposite to the one the person held. For example, a person who is opposed to abortion might believe that items presented on a survey represent a proabortion stance. A person who agrees to a telephone interview on political attitudes might find during questioning that the items seem slanted toward one political party. In this case, the person's neutral attitude might shift negatively, resulting in extreme negative responses. Likewise, students who are asked to complete an evaluation of an instructor after learning that they failed an exam are likely to approach the evaluation with considerable negativity. In this case, respondents might overreport negative attitudes.

To minimize the tendency to respond in either a satisfising or a negative manner, the researcher has available a number of strategies to motivate participants to do their best. High on this list is developing rapport with participants. The strategies for developing rapport vary depending on the interview situation. In a face-to-face interview, the interviewer can greet participants in a pleasant manner, begin the conversation with small talk, explain the study in an easy-to-understand manner, and show respect for participants. During the interview, the interviewer can use comments such as "You're doing a great job," and, "We're almost finished," to provide continued encouragement for the participant. Mail-out surveys can establish rapport through a letter to participants and through the formatting of the questionnaire. Other motivational techniques include carefully explaining the study to participants so that they know their role in responding to items. We assist participants by explaining the importance of this role in gathering accurate data and by instructing them to consider each item carefully before answering. Showing appreciation of the time and effort participants expend in completing the survey is important. In addition to using motivational techniques to gain their cooperation, keeping the task simple makes it easier for it to be completed in a timely manner. Researchers should use short items with easy-to-understand words, easy-to-follow directions, and clear formatting to reduce respondent burden (Streiner & Norman, 1995).

Response Sets. In studying the ways in which people respond to items, researchers have identified several patterns of responses, referred to as *response sets* or *bias*. Pedhazur and Schmelkin (1991, p. 140) define *response set* as "the tendency to provide responses independent of item content." Sometimes people are aware that they are responding to items in a biased manner, but more often, people are unconscious of their biases. Researchers have identified several different response sets, including social desirability, acquiescence, end aversion, positive skew, and halo.

Social Desirability. Edwards (1957) defined social desirability as "the tendency of subjects to attribute to themselves in self-description personality statements with socially desirable scale values and to reject those with socially undesirable scale values" (p. vi). In Edwards's description, people exhibiting a social desirability response set are more likely than most people to agree strongly with statements about their own good character, willingness to help others in all situations, refraining from lying, and friendly disposition. In health behavior research, people displaying this response set are more likely to agree strongly with statements associated with healthy behavior and disagree with statements suggesting unhealthy behavior. That is, people may strongly agree with statements that health is important to them (for example, "I exercise every day no matter what") and disagree with statements that might indicate poor health choices (for example, "I never read food labels"). People who intentionally try to create a favorable impression of themselves (as opposed to having an unconscious tendency to do so) exhibit a response set of faking goodness (Edwards, 1957). Thus, people who seek approval for being physically healthy may intentionally overestimate the amount of exercise they engage in each week or underestimate the amount of fat in their diets. For example, a person who does not eat many fruits and vegetables may indicate on a survey that he or she eats five fruits or vegetables per day based on his or her knowledge of the recommended amount. Likewise, someone who fails to exercise may respond that he or she does work out because he or she knows a person should do so to stay healthy.

The opposite of *faking good* is *faking bad*. A person who believes that portraying himself or herself in a negative way may be advantageous in a certain situation may answer items in a socially undesirable manner. For example, sometimes people choose to refrain from disclosing health behaviors that may make them less attractive for a research study. A woman who wants to participate in a research study that includes sessions with a personal trainer may fail to admit to regular exercise when in fact exercise is an important part of her life. Or a man who maintains good control of his diabetes may claim he finds it difficult to manage his disease so that he can participate in a study that offers a number of incentives.

Researchers can use several methods to reduce the tendency of participants to choose socially desirable answers. Participants who feel they can trust the researcher and believe in the confidentiality of the study are more likely to answer items truthfully. The researcher has an obligation to create an environment in which the respondent will feel comfortable, particularly when the researcher requests sensitive information (for example, "I have sex with more than one partner without using a condom"). To create an environment of trust, the researcher should provide adequate information about the study and explain how the data will be used. By mentioning that there are no right or wrong answers and that the data will be carefully secured, the researcher gives participants permission to respond as they truly feel.

To assess the extent to which social desirability may have influenced responses to a specific set of items, the researcher can correlate scores with a measure of social desirability. Crowne and Marlow (1960) developed one of the more popular social desirability scales, which contains items requiring a *yes* or *no* answer. Most people are likely to respond *yes* to at least some of the items on the scale, such as, "I have sometimes told a lie." Researchers believe that people who select mostly negative answers to this set of items are more likely to respond in a socially desirable manner to other items, including those of interest to the researcher. If scores on the items of interest are strongly correlated with scores on the social desirability scale, we can conclude that at least some respondents answered in a socially desirable manner. Because researchers usually collect data on the scale of interest to the researcher and the social desirability scale at the same time, the researcher must provide an interpretation based on these findings. A limitation of this type of study may be that the results reflect, to some extent, social desirability.

Acquiescence and Nay-Saying. Cronbach (1946) first identified the tendency of individuals to choose *true* over *false* in test taking (*true-saying*). The concept has expanded to include the tendency to select *agree* over *disagree* in Likert scales (*yea-saying*) and the tendency to choose *yes* over *no* (*yes-saying*) in dichotomous items (Couch & Keniston, 1960). Individuals who display this type of response set have a tendency to agree with both favorable and unfavorable statements, or to answer *true* to any statement. In response to items on healthy eating habits, a person exhibiting the acquiescence response set would tend to answer *yes* to items regardless of content. Acquiescence often leads to inconsistent responses. For example, a person might respond *yes* to indicate that he or she eats fruits five times per day and later respond *yes* to an item stating that he or she eats no more than three fruits per day. The opposite tendency also exists, where respondents are more likely to disagree than agree, choose *false* rather than *true*, or say *no* rather than *yes*. We refer to this pattern as *nay-saying.* The same type of inconsistent response is possible with the nay-saying response set. A questionnaire on smoking might have two items, one in which a person indicates that he or she would not allow someone to smoke in the house, and a second in which he or she indicates that he or she would not ask someone to go outside to smoke. Someone exhibiting the nay-saying response set would answer *no* to both items, leading to inconsistent responses.

End Aversion (Central Tendency). End aversion is a type of response set noted in items for which there are more than two response options (Streiner & Norman, 1995). Rating scales give people a choice of responses whose number is most often between three and ten. People who exhibit end aversion tend to avoid selection of extreme values on the rating scale. Thus, on a five-point rating scale, they would select neither one nor five. Likewise, on a ten-point rating scale, they would avoid one and ten. When interpreted, these responses indicate that these respondents fail to hold strong views on the topic. They are more likely to select an *agree* rather than a *strongly agree* response or a *disagree* rather than a *strongly disagree* response. Or they are more likely to note that they do something *most of the time* or *sometimes* rather than *always* or *never.* A particular type of end aversion involves selecting the middle category for all items. Thus, if the rating scale has an uneven number of choices (three, five, seven, or nine), the middle category will be selected (for example, three on a five-point rating scale). The best approach to minimize end aversion is to encourage participants to select from the full range of choices. In a face-to-face interview, the interviewer may provide this encouragement, or on a written questionnaire, the researcher can include this encouragement in the instructions.

Positive Skew. In some cases, people tend to hold extreme positive or negative attitudes about a topic (Streiner & Norman, 1995). As a result, they are likely to select the extreme rating choice—for example, *strongly agree* or *strongly disagree*—for all items. This response set differs from that of acquiescence and nay-saying. With acquiescence and nay-saying, there is a tendency to answer in the affirmative (or negative) regardless of item content. In the positive skew response set, content matters. The positive skew response set is manifested more with some attitudes and beliefs than with others. For example, people tend to rate their self-efficacy for a variety of behaviors very high—often seven or more on a ten-point scale. One strategy to control for positive skew is to examine the item content and modify (or tone) the wording to make it more difficult for someone to select an extreme value (Viswanathan, 2005). For example, the developer could add the term *always* in the stem of each item (for example, "I can always take my medicine at the same time each day"). Another strategy is to include items that assess the highest difficulty level (for example, "I can run an ultra marathon—100 miles"). Finally, providing a *very extreme* response category or providing more gradations (or options) of responses at one end of the scale can discourage extreme response choices. This last method is shown in Figure 3.1. Response Option A is a traditional Likert scale. If responses are skewed

FIGURE 3.1. RESPONSE OPTIONS.

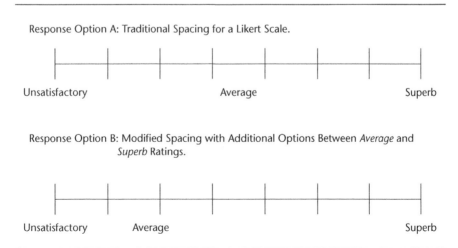

Response Option A: Traditional Spacing for a Likert Scale.

Unsatisfactory   Average   Superb

Response Option B: Modified Spacing with Additional Options Between *Average* and *Superb* Ratings.

Unsatisfactory   Average   Superb

Source: Steiner and Norman, 1995, p. 80. Reprinted by permission of Oxford University Press.

toward the *Superb* end of the scale, most of the responses will be found at the far right of the scale. However, if the center is shifted to the left, as in Response Option B, the respondent has more choices between the responses *Average* and *Superb*.

Halo. The halo effect is the tendency for ratings of specific traits to be influenced by a general attitude, or set, toward a person (Cooper, 1981). Halo effects are noted commonly in situations in which a rater is required to evaluate selected characteristics of an individual. Halo ratings occur when the rater allows a general attitude toward the person being evaluated to influence the rating of specific characteristics. For example, at the end of a course, students are usually asked to evaluate the instructor. Students might give an instructor whom they like high positive ratings on a set of course evaluation items regardless of how well certain aspects of the course were implemented. Also, an instructor might overestimate the ability of students who participate the most in class and give them higher grades than the ones they earned. In clinical settings, where instructors rate students on performance abilities, they might reward students who are well liked with higher ratings than they give to reserved students who are less inclined to seek attention from the instructor. The opposite of the halo effect is the pitchfork effect, in which a general negative impression of a person influences ratings of specific characteristics (Lowe, 1986). Thus, an instructor who is less engaging might receive lower ratings, without justification, on specific characteristics of the course.

Cooper (1981), who studied the halo response set extensively, gives nine ways in which investigators can reduce the halo effect. The strategies most useful for health behavior researchers include training evaluators regarding ways to rate participants, taking steps to ensure consistency across raters, and having evaluators record critical incidences to use as justification for their ratings. Evaluators who are familiar with the participants are more likely to be aware of the full range of behaviors that the participants might exhibit, and that they in turn would evaluate. For example, having a professor for more than one class allows the student to see that teacher function in different contexts, thus increasing the likelihood of an accurate evaluation.

Recall. In addition to response sets, a major source of measurement error in self-report instruments is related to the ability and motivation of respondents to provide accurate information about behaviors or events that have occurred in the past. When responding to items that require the recollection of information from memory, participants often feel pressure to respond immediately after a question is asked or read. Unless they are instructed otherwise by the interviewer, the respondents tend to answer relatively quickly even though the requested information requires recall and calculation components. For example, when asked, "How many times did you eat fruit last week?" a respondent generally would not take the time to search his or her memory for the exact days on which fruit was eaten and then calculate how much was consumed each day during the week. This recall and calculation process would take some time. Thus, the most common response is a quick estimation of fruit intake based on general experience. In these situations, a process called *telescoping* often occurs, in which respondents include more events within a time period than they should.

There are a number of ways in which investigators can enhance recall of past events. The cognitive interview is one such method used by health professionals to enhance recall of health-related behaviors and events. Fisher and Quigley (1992) developed the cognitive interview to enhance recall of food consumption. Their work was based on the need to trace the sources of food-borne illnesses. When food-borne illness outbreaks occur, epidemiologists depend on affected people to provide accurate and complete recall of foods they have eaten within the past two to seven days. However, studies using standard interview questions reveal that errors in food consumption recall are common (Decker, Booth, et al., 1986; Mann, 1981). The cognitive interview is based on five principles of cognition and memory retrieval: (1) context reinstatement, (2) focused retrieval, (3) extensive retrieval, (4) varied retrieval, and (5) multiple representations. Using the principle of context reinstatement, Fisher and Quigley asked people to think about environmental conditions (for example, room, lighting, people present) and psychological context (for example, reason for selecting the food) when they ate a meal. To recall events, people need to be able to retrieve information from memory (focused retrieval). To encourage them to do so, the investigators allowed people to think without interruptions or distractions, and they encouraged the respondents to take their time in performing this task. The principles of extensive and varied retrieval suggest that the more attempts one makes and the more varied the attempts, the more successful one will be in recalling food eaten. Thus, the investigators asked people to continue to search their memories even after they said they could remember no more. To make this task less redundant, the investigators varied the questions. For example, a direct question, such as "Did you have mayonnaise on your sandwich?" would later be followed by the request, "Tell me what was on your sandwich." The multiple-representation principle is based on the idea that images of an event are stored in different forms and asking about these different images may elicit new information. Food images might include food on the plate, food carried by the waiter, and food shared with others. Information from Fisher and Quigley's studies indicates that retrieval of information and accuracy are greater using the cognitive interview than using standard interview questions.

This approach has its disadvantages. The most significant is the amount of time it takes to conduct a cognitive interview. In their study, Fisher and Quigley noted that the cognitive interview took an average of 15 minutes and the interview with standard questions an average of 1.5 minutes. The cognitive interview is also unsuitable for the written questionnaire. The investigator might include specific instructions on a questionnaire asking a person to be mindful of the context of a situation and spend some time remembering the event. However, the investigator has no way of knowing whether the respondent followed the instructions.

The cognitive-interview approach has been modified for use in collecting other health-related data, including risky sexual practices, medication taking, and food consumption during the past twenty-four hours. For example, Chesney and colleagues (2000) developed the AACTG medication adherence measure, which includes an interview with participants concerning the number of medications missed during the past four days. Participants are first asked to consider the preceding day and to think carefully about taking their medications, including the number, types, and contexts of the medication-taking events. After participants complete that task, the day before yesterday is considered; the sequence is continued until all four days have been reviewed.

Instrument Factors

Another major component of measurement error is associated with the instrument itself. Some instrument factors that tend to increase error are:

- Inadequate instructions
- Poor formatting
- Illogical order of items
- Use of vague or unfamiliar terms
- Response options that vary
- Items that fail to correspond to the scale
- Response options that fail to fit the question
- Items that favor one group over another
- Equipment that is not properly maintained or calibrated

If anyone needs to be convinced that measurement instruments can themselves account for a significant portion of error, such a person need only consider the "butterfly ballot" of the 2000 presidential election in Florida. Palm Beach County election officials designed the ballot to list candidates' names on both the right and left sides of the ballot. To choose a candidate whose name appeared on the left, voters had to punch the circle to the right of his or her name. To choose a candidate whose name appeared on the right, voters had to punch the circle to the left of his or her name. The circles appeared in a vertical line down the center of the ballot. The ballot was confusing for several reasons, but the most frequent complaint was confusion about the placement of candidate Al Gore's name. The second name on the left side of the ballot was Al Gore, but the second circle down corresponded to the name of candidate Pat Buchanan, the first name on the right side of the ballot. Many people punched the second circle in the belief that they were voting for Al Gore, when in fact their votes went to Pat Buchanan.

We can find similar problems on written questionnaires designed to collect data on health behaviors. Consider the quiz on HIV knowledge presented in Exhibit 3.1. Note that one of the problems with the quiz is the absence of instructions. Although most people would probably know how to answer the *true* and *false* items without instructions, responding to items on the lower part of the quiz would be difficult without some direction. The semantic differential scale is not a common method of collecting data, and without instructions, people are likely to skip the section or respond according to their own interpretations of the task. Other errors on the quiz include misspelled words (for example, *changes* instead of *chances)*, poor formatting, and undefined terms (CD4 counts). Respondents who score poorly on this quiz would be classified as having a low level of knowledge about HIV. However, if their errors were due to problems with the quiz itself, the results would lead to false conclusions about HIV knowledge.

In recent years, computer-assisted interviewing (CAI) has become a popular method of collecting data because of savings in interviewer and data entry time. By having participants enter their own responses to items directly into the computer, errors due to ambiguous responses (for example, circling two response options on a survey) and those due to faulty data entry are reduced. Despite these advantages, CAI generates its own type of errors, which the user must consider. In our own experience with using CAI, especially early versions of the software, we found that some responses

EXHIBIT 3.1. EXAMPLE OF A KNOWLEDGE TEST DEMONSTRATING INSTRUMENT-RELATED ERRORS.

HIV KNOWLEDGE TEST

A person can get HIV if he or she has unprotected sexual intercourse.	True	False
A person get HIV if he or she shares a needle with someone.	True	False
A person can reduce his or her changes of getting HIV if he uses a condom.	True	False
A person can get HIV from a blood transfusion.	True	False
A person with a very low CD4 count can run a marathon. False		True

MY KNOWLEDGE OF HIV IS

Good	___	___	___	___	___	___	___	Bad
Fast	___	___	___	___	___	___	___	Slow
Strong	___	___	___	___	___	___	___	Weak
Active	___	___	___	___	___	___	___	Passive

were missing at random or whole sections of surveys were not saved properly. Programmed instructions to skip selected items did not always function properly, and some items were skipped for no apparent reason. Files were not saved properly due to a variety of factors, including software and hardware problems and interviewer errors. Developers of the software continually work to address these problems, but researchers must be mindful that problems do exist and set up protocols to check data immediately after the questionnaire is completed by the respondent.

Another instrument factor that health educators and behavioral scientists must consider is poorly maintained equipment. Monitors designed to measure blood pressure, heart rate, weight, oxygen consumption, and other health variables need to be calibrated periodically and properly maintained according to the manufacturers' directions. Failure to do so may lead to false readings, which can in turn affect the results of the study or evaluation.

Strategies to Reduce Errors on Self-Report Questionnaires. Because measurement error is likely to affect all types of self-report instruments, the researcher should be aware of ways to reduce measurement error. Dillman (Salant & Dillman, 1994; Dillman, 2000) has written extensively on survey design, providing a variety of helpful strategies to engage the participant in the research while avoiding mistakes that lead to incorrect or inaccurate responses. In the Tailored Design Method, researchers pay attention to the introduction of the study (either in a written cover letter for paper-and-pencil and mail surveys or in the introductory patter for in-person and telephone surveys). A thoughtful and engaging introduction can determine whether or not a person agrees to participate in the study and can also affect the mental attitude (optimizing, satisfising, or negative) of the person when he or she is completing the survey. The presentation of the survey, in areas such as the study title, the front cover of the survey, and the format, affects a person's initial impression. A survey that lacks an appealing title and includes numerous questions on each page with little space between items is less engaging than one with a catchy title, an appealing front cover, and an interesting format. Moreover, tightly spaced questions can cause response errors. To hold the attention of the participant, Dillman also suggests beginning the survey with items relevant to the survey and placing the demographic items at the end of the survey. Researchers should place any sensitive items about halfway through the survey. The researcher can help participants by providing transitions (for example, "In the next section, you will be asked questions about . . .") and placing the instructions for answering each set of items above the items rather than at the beginning of the interview or in the cover letter. Other strategies to reduce respondent error include using arrows to link questions when an item is skipped, keeping the format simple, using a legible type size, and providing mutually exclusive and exhaustive answer choices. Finally, researchers should carefully edit and pretest the survey with a sample of participants similar to those for whom they designed the instrument. Many of these strategies can be used in the development of computer-based interviews as well.

Strategies to Reduce Errors During Interviews. According to Pedhazur and Schmelkin (1991, p. 134), "interviewer effects are inevitable." The primary concern of the researcher is to identify the types of interviewer effects that exist and to employ strategies for reducing errors and minimizing their effects on the data. Interviewer errors can include, but are not limited to, failing to read the items as written, skipping items, using inappropriate probes, providing inconsistent feedback, recording responses inaccurately, leading participants to respond in a specific manner, and failing to maintain an environment conducive to a successful interview. In addition to errors made by the interviewer, characteristics of the interviewer can influence the way a participant responds. Gender, age, race, and socioeconomic background are the characteristics that investigators have studied the most in this regard. The literature provides some evidence that the attitudes and opinions of interviewers can be reflected in the participants' responses (Erdos, 1970; Pedhazur & Schmelkin, 1991). To reduce interviewer effects, training is essential. Training should include, at the very least, the protocols for the interview and the questionnaire. During training, interviewers learn about the purpose of the study and the importance of collecting accurate and complete data. They have numerous opportunities to practice the questionnaire, including the speed of reading items, probing for additional information, providing feedback, and completing the questionnaire forms.

Situational Factors

A third component of measurement error is associated with the situation in which the measurement of the concept is taking place or at the point of data analysis. Some situational factors that might tend to induce or increase error are:

*   Environment (heat, cold, noise, rain)
*   Concurrent or past events (9/11)
*   Chance events
*   Administration errors
*   Time factors
*   Investigator errors
*   Scoring errors

Returning to our Florida example, the 2000 presidential election provides an excellent example of factors that influenced the scoring of responses (votes). A point of contention for that election was the manner in which pollsters counted (or scored) votes.

To count the votes by hand, the county canvassing boards had to decide how to read the measuring instrument (the ballot) and then determine which of the following would count as a vote (*chads* are the small pieces of paper punched or partly punched out of a ballot):

- Hanging chad
- Dimpled chad
- Pregnant chad
- Three-cornered chad
- Dimpled chad for presidential vote, but clean votes for other offices
- Dimpled chad for all votes
- Two votes for the same office
- Mark other than a stylus mark on the chad (fingernail, pencil, or pen)
- Light visible through the margins of the chad.

Here, the problem lay not with the respondent or the instrument, but with the voting process and the scoring. In some cases, voting officials failed to provide clear instructions on how to ensure that a vote actually was cast, because electronic counting machines can count only votes without chads. The decisions for counting each of the conditions listed previously as a vote varied among counties and sometimes within a county.

What would happen if we applied the same approach to the Graduate Record Examination (GRE)? Would an examination with no consistent rules for scoring be considered reliable? Or valid? Chances are that we would consider an examination without standard, explicit, and unambiguous rules for scoring to be unreliable or invalid, and as a result, graduate schools would refuse to use the results for important decisions regarding admission to their programs.

To calculate scores that provide a fair and objective representation of how well students do on the GRE, the developers must make decisions or rules about scoring the examination. We can think of a student's total score on the exam as the measure of the general fund of knowledge the student possesses at the time of taking the exam. In generating the score, or the empirical measure of knowledge, the developers must develop rules for each of the following:

- How each correct response will be scored
- How each incorrect response will be scored
- How a skipped item will be scored
- How an item with more than one answer will be scored
- How many correct items will correspond to the overall score

Beyond scoring issues, there are a variety of situational factors that can influence the measurement of health-related variables. The types of situational factors will depend on the variables themselves and on the instrument used to measure the variables. When blood samples are collected, for example, blood for some tests must be kept at room temperature and blood for other tests must be refrigerated. Failure to keep the blood at the proper temperature can affect the results. Likewise, appropriate reagents are needed in conducting various tests of bodily functions. Using the wrong reagents will lead to false scores. Investigator errors might include failure to reverse score items on a scale or using the wrong items to compute a scale score.

Measurement Rules. One of the most important ways in which we can avoid situational errors is to provide a clear set of rules for each measurement instrument. Nunnally and Bernstein (1994) note that procedures for assigning numbers to characteristics of an object must be standardized, explicit, unambiguous, and subject to evaluation. The measurement process must be standardized so that it is applied in the same way each time the instrument is administered. The rules should be explicit so that any person using the instrument uses it in the same manner as others. The rules must be clear and apply to all possible uses of the instrument. Rules that are ambiguous will yield different results because of uncertainty as to how to use the instrument or how to score it. Finally, we should subject the rules to evaluation, so that after use, we can make modifications in the scoring rules if necessary. Although the developer usually creates rules for the use of a measuring device, a rule might need to be changed with the experience of using the instrument over time.

Summary

Error is an inevitable but undesirable component of measurement. Error affects the reliability and validity of scores and, if severe, can lead to flawed interpretation of the data. Errors are generally classified as random or systematic; random errors influence reliability more, and systematic ones have a greater effect on validity. The factors that create errors in measurement can be broadly classified as those due to respondent, instrument, and situational factors. Respondent errors have received considerable attention in the literature and a number of strategies have been suggested to reduce respondents' errors, including those due to response biases and faulty recall of information. Likewise, an extensive literature also speaks to techniques for reducing errors attributed to characteristics of the instrument and to factors arising during and after the measurement process. In Chapters Nine, Ten, and Eleven, we will build on the information presented here in our discussion of reliability and validity assessment.

CHAPTER FOUR

SURVEY DEVELOPMENT

LEARNING OBJECTIVES

At the end of this chapter, the student should be able to

1. Describe the characteristics of a survey.
2. Discuss the basic principles of survey construction.
3. Apply the principles of item writing.
4. Revise poorly written items.
5. Describe the association between item wording and measurement error.
6. Describe the association between survey format and measurement error.
7. Discuss four methods of survey administration.

In the course of their work, health educators and behavioral scientists often construct surveys to collect information about a variety of health-related topics. Consider Daniel, who works as the infection control coordinator at a large metropolitan hospital center. Recently, several units experienced an outbreak of staphylococcus infection after years of very low infection rates. In addition to collecting specimens from the affected units and conducting a thorough cleaning of rooms and equipment, Daniel has also developed a survey. His objective was to determine the current hand-hygiene practices of unit personnel and to find out the extent to which they use the new hand-cleansing agents adopted by the hospital within the past year. Daniel plans to survey hospital personnel working on three intensive care units, on five medical and surgical units, and in three outpatient clinics that have reported infections within the past six months. Daniel realizes that the construction of a good survey will take time and must incorporate specific steps (outlined later in Figure 4.1).

Though the primary focus of this book is on scale development and testing, we have included this chapter to acquaint students with survey development and the essentials of item writing. We begin with a definition of a survey and then present brief descriptions of the six components necessary to the development of a useful survey: purpose, objectives, respondents, items, format, and administration. This description is not intended to be a complete course in survey development. However, it will raise awareness of the issues involved in survey development and the difference between surveys and scales.

Definition

Surveys are self-report instruments used by researchers and others to gather information on a variety of issues. Health behavior researchers use surveys to collect data on health behaviors or the variety of factors associated with health behaviors. Public health professionals rely on surveys to explore people's knowledge, attitudes, beliefs, and behaviors; to ask about feelings and opinions; and to collect personal information about respondents. Surveys offer a convenient and efficient way to collect self-report data. Moreover, survey developers find the responses generally easy to record, and data relatively easy to enter and analyze. Surveys, particularly anonymous surveys, allow researchers to collect information on sensitive topics, ranging from age and income to risky sexual behaviors.

Basic Principles of Survey Construction

Purpose

The development of a survey begins with a broad statement of its purpose (Figure 4.1). Although this fact seems obvious, it is easy to lose focus when developing a survey and end up with a product that lacks integrity. Take, for example, a group of health behavior researchers participating in a research project designed to examine factors related to self-management in persons with epilepsy. As part of the study, the researchers planned to collect background information to describe the participants in the study. They planned to include items such as age, gender, education, and information about seizure history and medication use. The researchers also wanted to know about a number of

FIGURE 4.1. STEPS IN SURVEY DEVELOPMENT.

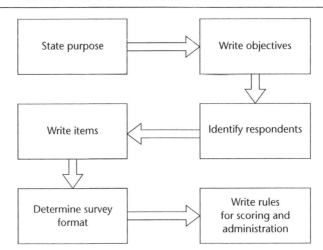

other issues, including how long participants had been treated for epilepsy, sources of information, types of insurance, and confidence in the health care system, among other things. They wrote items to collect information on these topics as well as the usual background information. Before long, the background section of the survey extended to fifty-five items, many of which were unrelated to the primary purpose of describing the sample. When the researchers realized it would take participants as much time to complete the background section as the items on self-management, they deleted most of the new items. The researchers could have saved considerable time if they had started with a clear statement of purpose.

Objectives

After researchers determine the general purpose of the survey, they list specific objectives or research questions to guide them in the development of actual survey items. For example, a broad statement of purpose for a survey of hand-hygiene practices of unit personnel in acute care settings might be as follows: *to collect information about hand-hygiene practices of unit personnel in acute care settings.* Asking one question, such as "Do you wash your hands before caring for each patient?" might be insufficient to address the broad purpose. Daniel, as noted earlier, also wants to know how often unit personnel wash their hands each day, whether or not they have developed contact dermatitis, and what they perceive as barriers to hand-hygiene practices. He is also interested in the types of agents personnel use to clean their hands and the use of alternative practices, such as wearing gloves. Finally, Daniel might also want to know how important unit personnel think hand washing is. To meet all his objectives, he will need to include specific questions addressing each of these aims. Thus, for his hand-hygiene survey, Daniel might list the following research questions:

- How often do unit personnel wash their hands before caring for a patient?
- How often do unit personnel use soap and water or antiseptic agents when washing their hands?
- How often do unit personnel use both antiseptic agents and water when washing their hands?
- How often do unit personnel use alcohol-based hand rubs, instead of soap and water or antiseptic agents with water, to clean their hands?
- What percentage of unit personnel have developed irritant contact dermatitis due to frequent hand-hygiene practices?
- What are the perceived barriers to performing hand-hygiene practices?
- How important do unit personnel believe it is to wash their hands?

The research questions guide the selection of items for inclusion in the survey (Exhibit 4.1). The more specific the research questions, the easier it is to select items. Research questions that are broad or vague make the selection of items difficult.

Purpose and Research Questions for a Survey of Students' Attitudes About Exercise

For a study of the exercise habits of college students, a researcher might state the following purpose and ask the following research questions.

Purpose: To examine college students' attitudes toward, and participation in, various forms of exercise.

Research Questions
- What percentage of college students exercise three or more times per week?
- What types of exercises or sports do college students participate in?
- What do students believe are the benefits of exercise?
- How confident are students that they can exercise three or more times per week under varying conditions?

EXHIBIT 4.1. EXAMPLE OF SURVEY ITEMS ON HAND-HYGIENE PRACTICES.

Please answer the following questions about your hand-hygiene practices.

What type of unit do you work on?

1. _____ Inpatient floor
2. _____ Intensive care unit
3. _____ Operating room
4. _____ Outpatient unit

About how often do you wash your hands *every hour*?

1. _____ 0–1 time
2. _____ 2–4 times
3. _____ 5–7 times
4. _____ 9–10 times
5. _____ More than 10 times

How often do you wash your hands before caring for a patient?

1. _____ Every time
2. _____ Most of the time
3. _____ Sometimes
4. _____ Hardly ever
5. _____ Never

How often do you use soap or antiseptic agents when washing your hands?

1. _____ Every time
2. _____ Most of the time
3. _____ Sometimes
4. _____ Hardly ever
5. _____ Never

Have you ever developed irritant contact dermatitis due to frequent hand-hygiene practices?

1. _____ Yes
2. _____ No
3. _____ Not sure

Which of the following reasons prevent you from performing hand-hygiene practices? (Check all that apply)

1. _____ Hand-washing agents cause irritation.
2. _____ Soap or paper towels are not provided.
3. _____ I wear gloves.
4. _____ Sinks are not conveniently located.

Respondents

The next step in developing a survey is to consider the respondents:

- Who are the respondents?
- What are their expected levels of language and reading skills?
- How familiar are they with the topic?
- How will respondents be recruited for the study?
- How much time will they have to complete the survey?
- Will they be willing to respond to the survey?

Young children with limited reading and writing skills would need an interviewer to read questions to them, as would adult respondents with poor literacy or physical limitations that interfere with reading or writing. If the researcher believes some respondents might be unfamiliar with the topic, definitions of some terms should be provided.

Just as the researchers assessing epilepsy self-management made decisions about what to include in the epilepsy background information survey, researchers must make tough decisions about the inclusion of survey items based on the amount of time available. If the respondents have only five minutes, ten to fifteen questions may be the maximum number that they can answer.

Nurses and other professionals working on hospital units tend to be extremely busy. Therefore, our public health professionals who want to ask them to complete a survey on hand-hygiene practices must bear in mind the respondents' time restrictions when developing their survey. A short survey, such as that presented in Exhibit 4.1, would probably take a few minutes to complete, and nurses might be willing to complete it during the course of their work day. This survey would be useful to gather preliminary information that could be used to develop a more comprehensive questionnaire on hand-hygiene practices.

General Principles of Item Writing

After the purpose and objectives are clearly stated and the respondent issues are identified, the next step in survey development is to write the items that correspond to the objectives. There are several approaches that can be used to write items. One approach is to rephrase the objectives and add the appropriate response options. Before this is done, however, some general principles of survey development and item writing are important to understand.

The first principle of survey development is related to the respondents' process of completing the survey. Clark and Schober (1994) note that what appears to be a simple process of providing information on the survey is actually a complex interaction. They make clear that it is important for the researcher to think about a survey in terms of an exchange of information between a researcher and a respondent. In the simplest exchange, the respondent first reads and then answers the survey items. Understanding both the role of the researcher's intentions in asking the questions and the meaning attributed to the questions by the respondent is important in developing high-quality items that minimize measurement error.

In a normal conversation, people develop a common ground, or common understanding of the discussion (Clark & Schober, 1994). Generally, conversation consists of the logical progression of ideas and information, strung together by the contributions of each participant in a discussion. Speakers make statements in such a way that the people to whom they speak can understand what they are saying. Unless a respondent requests clarification, we assume that the recipients of the speaker's statements understand what is being said. As the conversation moves along, topics change, but those who are paying attention to the conversation realize it has headed in a different direction.

In an ordinary conversation, participants in the discussion contribute in real time. However, with a survey, one participant in the conversation, the researcher, writes all the questions before the respondent ever answers the first one. Thus, the challenge for the researcher is to build the common ground for the survey, which includes making statements clear so that respondents know how to answer each question and providing sufficient instructions for the completion of the survey along with directions for changes in the topics within the survey. Using these principles of language along with some common prescriptions for item writing, we present some do's and don'ts for writing items. These suggestions are based on the work of several authors who have studied the art and science of asking questions (Sudman & Bradburn, 1982; Dillman, 2000).

The Do's of Item Writing

1. Write items that are related to the purpose of the survey and that address the objectives. When participants are told the purpose of the survey, they will expect to answer questions that are related to the topic (Dillman, 2000). That is, the items should reflect the purpose of the survey and be transparent to the respondent. If the purpose of the survey is to identify the exercise habits of college students, a respondent will not expect to see items about attitudes toward instructors. If the researchers include items that are not transparent, they should tell the participants how these items are related to the study. For example, if a researcher is interested in familial and peer factors associated with exercise, some items are likely to refer to the exercise habits of friends and family members. A simple statement at the beginning of the study telling the participant that the study will also examine how others influence their exercise habits helps participants understand the rationale for these questions.

2. Write each item as a complete sentence with a subject and a verb. Typically, people who are conversing speak in complete sentences rather than single words or short phrases.

> *Weak:* Age_____
>
> *Revision:* What is your age?_____

3. Write items that are short and concise when requesting information about neutral topics. Short questions are easier for respondents to read. Longer questions take more time to read and are subject to more error if the respondent fails to read the items carefully and responds inappropriately. In addition, long questions are likely to include more than one idea, making it difficult for the respondent to answer.

> *Weak:* Do you ever eat fruits and vegetables that are not washed because you don't have time to wash them or because you don't think that unwashed fruits and vegetables are harmful?
>
> Yes_____ No_____
>
> *Revision:* Do you wash fruits and vegetables before you eat them?
>
> Yes_____ No_____
>
> If no, which of the following are your reasons for not washing them? (Check all that apply.)
>
> _____ Not enough time
>
> _____ Not concerned about harmful bacteria
>
> _____ Habit

Sometimes participants need background information about a topic before encountering the questions. This background information may make the question seem very long. In this case, separating the information from the question helps the respondent see exactly what is being asked.

People with epilepsy may have different types of seizures. The two primary types are generalized seizures and partial seizures. Generalized seizures always involve loss of consciousness and can involve movements of all extremities. Partial seizures may include loss of consciousness; however, movements or sensations are usually limited to one part of the body.

> Would you say that your most recent seizure was a generalized seizure or a partial seizure?
>
> _____ Generalized
>
> _____ Partial

4. Write open-ended or long items when requesting information about sensitive topics.

People tend to underreport occurrences of socially undesirable behaviors and overreport occurrences of socially desirable behaviors. Sensitive behaviors, such as drug and alcohol use and sexual and criminal behaviors, are likely to be underreported, whereas healthy behaviors are likely to be overreported. Sudman and Bradburn (1982) suggest using open-ended questions and longer questions when asking about threatening or sensitive behaviors.

Respondents often infer from response alternatives that the researcher knows what is normal and is presenting them with response options within the normal range. People reporting on sensitive behaviors may want to appear to fall within the normal range, so they may choose a middle response option. The provision of response alternatives can encourage underreporting or overreporting of some behaviors. In the example given here, we might interpret a history of six sexual partners as the upper limit of normality. However, a person who has had eight partners might select a response of 1–2 or 3–5 to appear to be within the normal range.

> *Weak:* How many sexual partners have you had in your lifetime?
>
> _____ None
>
> _____ 1–2
>
> _____ 3–5
>
> _____ 6 or more

> *Revision:* How many sexual partners have you had in your lifetime? _____

Loading is another way to encourage accurate responses for both open- and closed-ended questions (Sudman & Bradburn, 1982). Before asking the actual question, the researcher places the behavior in a context that encourages the participant to report behavior occurrences accurately. In the following example, the loaded statement lets the participant know that having sex without a condom is common.

Not loaded: Did you use a condom the last time you had sex?

Yes_____ No_____

Loaded: Many times people want to use a condom, but they forget or they don't have one with them, and so they have sex without a condom. Did you use a condom the last time you had sex?

Yes_____ No_____

Another approach is to use authority to justify behavior.

Recent studies suggest that drinking two or more cups of coffee with caffeine each day is good for your heart. How many cups of coffee with caffeine did you have yesterday? _____

5. *Write response choices that are mutually exclusive and exhaustive.* When respondents must make a choice in the selection of a response, the response set should include all possible choices. In addition, choices should be mutually exclusive, so that a respondent cannot select more than one.

Weak: What is your marital status?

_____ Single

_____ Married

_____ Living with a partner

_____ Divorced

Revision: What is your marital status?

_____ Married

_____ Never married

_____ Divorced

_____ Widowed

_____ Separated

Are you currently living with a partner?

Yes_____ No_____

If numerous possible response choices exist, a researcher may include several of the most common and then have a final choice labeled *other,* allowing the respondent the option of writing his or her response if it is unavailable on the list.

What is your religion?

1. _____ Buddhist
2. _____ Catholic
3. _____ Jewish
4. _____ Muslim
5. _____ Protestant
6. _____ Other (please specify) _____

6. *Spell out acronyms.* A search of acronyms on the Internet reveals that the same acronym may refer to many different organizations, programs, or ideas. For example, the American Medical Association and the Association of Media Agents both use *AMA* as an acronym. Individuals reading a question that contains an acronym are likely to interpret and thus respond to the question with their own particular understandings of what the acronym means to them. The same is true for abbreviations. If a survey needs an abbreviation throughout, the developers should define it first in the introductory section and use the full term in the first question.

Weak: Are you a member of APHA?

Revision: Are you a member of the American Public Health Association (APHA)?

Weak: Have you ever been tested for HIV?

Revision: Acquired immunodeficiency syndrome (AIDS) is caused by the human immunodeficiency virus (HIV). There is a simple blood test for HIV. Have you ever been tested for HIV?

Yes_____ No_____

7. *Define unusual terms.* Respondents seem to have stable opinions on issues about which they know nothing (Clark & Schober, 1994). Generally, respondents believe that if a researcher asks a question, they should understand what is being asked and will be able to answer the question. Thus, respondents will give opinions on issues about which they know little or nothing. Likewise, respondents tend to interpret vague words in the moment, choosing the closest meaning they can think of at that time; this often leads to inaccurate responses. In the weak item in the following example, respondents may believe that *vocational rehabilitation* refers to something akin to physical therapy and respond accordingly. If a vague term is necessary, the researchers should define it. A better approach is to select a term or phrase that is more descriptive of the concept presented.

Weak: Have you ever attended vocational rehabilitation?

Yes_____ No_____

Revision: Following your accident, have you attended sessions with a career counselor for job training?

Yes_____ No_____

8. Write items that contain one idea. If, during the course of a conversation, a speaker asks, "Do you think the Atkins and South Beach diets are good?" then others in the discussion may choose to respond by commenting on either one of the two diets or by providing a comparison. However, if investigators present an item that includes two ideas (also called a double-barreled item) in the context of a survey with forced-choice options, the respondent must decide how best to respond. If the respondent has a different opinion about each idea, he or she might choose a response based on one of the ideas or choose a response that seems to be on the middle ground.

For example, a respondent might find it difficult to answer the following weak question about helmet use for drivers and passengers because he or she always wears a helmet and his or her passengers never do. Because of potential differences in responses to the two ideas, the surveyor should present the ideas separately.

Weak: How often do you and your passengers wear helmets when you ride motorcycles?

Revision: How often do you wear a helmet when your ride a motorcycle?

and

How often do your passengers wear a helmet when they ride with you?

9. Write items that are specific. In developing items, the researcher needs to consider how people might respond to each item. An item that seems fairly simple to the researcher might generate confusion for the respondent. Consider the following question about drinking. In the weak example, the respondent might wonder what the researcher meant by the word *drink*. More often, the respondent assumes that the researcher would agree with the respondent's interpretation of the item. However, if the respondent thought that *drink* included only water, his or her response would be limited to the amount of water he or she drinks. Another respondent might believe that *drink* refers to alcoholic beverages only and answer accordingly. The researcher, however, might have wanted to learn about the full range of fluids an individual drinks in a day.

Weak: On average, how much do you drink per day?

Revision: On average, how many 8 ounce glasses of fluid do you drink each day? Include water, juice, coffee, tea, soft drinks, soups, and other liquids.

10. *Use simple words.* Survey development experts generally suggest that items be written at the sixth- through eighth-grade levels. To meet the criteria for these levels, items are generally short, with simple, common words. Researchers may dismiss this advice when they plan to survey college-educated individuals. However, even college graduates find it easier to read items written at a lower reading level, and the lower reading level makes the task easier and faster.

> *Weak:* How confident are you that you can differentiate eustress from distress in your daily life?
>
> *Revision:* How confident are you that you can tell the difference between things that encourage you to succeed and things that cause you stress in your daily life?

11. *Highlight terms that could easily be missed or that are particularly important.* In normal conversation, a speaker may emphasize a statement by changing the volume or quality of his or her voice. Written communication fulfills the same function through the use of capitals, boldface, italics, underlining, or color changes to draw attention to a word or a phrase. One word often missed in items is *not*. Therefore, if the survey includes items that contain the word *not* or prefixes such as *non-* and *un-*, the researcher should draw attention to them.

> *Weak:* When was the last time you did not take your medicines?
>
> *Revision:* When was the last time you did *not* take your medicines?

12. *For recall items, allow a specific time period that is consistent with the behavior.* In responding to items, participants feel pressure to respond as soon as a question has been asked or read. As in normal conversation, a person responds relatively quickly when asked a question, even if the question calls for information that requires recall and calculation. For example, when a respondent is asked in normal conversation, "How many times did you eat fruit last week?" he or she is usually not expected to actually take the time to recall exactly on which days fruit was eaten and how much. This process would take too long, so respondents give a quick estimate to provide an answer in a reasonable amount of time. When responding to a survey question, the participant also uses a process to quickly estimate the amount of fruit eaten last week, unless he or she is given instructions on how to estimate the amount. To minimize measurement error, researchers may provide respondents with a reasonable period of time that is consistent with the behavior. When asking about frequently occurring, routine behaviors, consider asking about the last day or the last week. For behaviors that occur less frequently or those that respondents are more likely to remember, the last month or the last year might be the most appropriate time frame.

Weak: How many fruits did you eat during the past week?

How many times have you visited the doctor in the past week?

Revision: How many fruits did you eat yesterday?

How many times have you visited the doctor in the past six months?

Additional ways to aid recall are to give specific dates and examples.

How many times have you been admitted to the hospital or treated in the emergency room since January 1, 2005?

How many college organizations, such as sororities, fraternities, political clubs, and foreign language groups, do you belong to?

13. *Use ranges rather than precise values for sensitive items.* When respondents reply to items about sensitive information, they are sometimes more likely to answer if they have a range of responses from which to select. This advice appears to conflict with rule 4, which suggests using open-ended questions to gather information about sensitive behavior. This example demonstrates that the researcher must understand the advantages and disadvantages of both approaches and make decisions based on the survey population and the goals of the research. In the case of income, people are much more likely to respond if they are given a range. The highest level of the range should be consistent with the population. For example, with middle-class and higher-income people, the upper range of household income might be $250,000 or more.

Weak: What was your total household income last year? _____

Revision: What was your total household income last year? (Please check one.)
_____ $0–19,999
_____ $20,000–39,999
_____ $40,000–59,999
_____ $60,000–79,999
_____ $80,000 or more

14. *Use response options such as* don't know *and* not applicable *sparingly.* One common decision researchers must make is whether to use a *don't know* category. Participants who are not offered *don't know* as an option will generally choose one of the categories that are presented. Only a few will indicate that they don't know when this option is not available. When *don't know* is offered, the percentage of respondents choosing this category is likely to increase.

No option given: HIV is caused by a virus.

True_____ False_____

Option given: HIV is caused by a virus.

True_____ False_____ Don't know_____

15. Make careful decisions about which response options to include. Questions with and without response alternatives imply different perspectives (Clark & Schober, 1994). The respondent generally assumes that the researcher wants a response consistent with the domains presented in the item and does not want the respondent to consider other areas. If the researcher asks a participant whether he or she likes to walk or run for exercise, the respondent will consider only these two options when replying. If, however, the researcher asks the respondent, "What do you like to do for exercise?" the respondent has a full range of choices.

Conversely, providing a list of alternatives may remind participants of responses that might not have occurred to them without prompting. For example, when asked what they like to do for exercise, most people will select *walking*. However, if they are given a list that includes activities such as gardening, a higher percentage of respondents are likely to select gardening.

Without response options: What is the most important health problem for people in the United States today? _____

With response options: What is the most important health problem for people in the United States today?

_____ Accidents

_____ AIDS

_____ Arthritis

_____ Asthma

_____ Cancer

_____ Diabetes

_____ Heart disease

_____ Obesity

The Don'ts of Item Writing

1. Don't write items that contain the word "not." Because respondents often miss the word *not* when they are reading items quickly, most measurement experts suggest phrasing an item to avoid using the word.

Weak: When was the last time you did not take your medications?

Revision: When was the last time you forgot to take your medications?

2. Don't write items that contain jargon or regional expressions. In the example below, Midwesterners would use the word *pop* to refer to carbonated beverages. Atlantans would use the word *Coke* for the same items, and in New Bern, North Carolina, the birthplace of Pepsi-Cola, the residents prefer the word *Pepsi* for carbonated beverages. Using a word with a regional meaning may be confusing to people from other parts of the country.

Weak: How many ounces of pop did you drink today? _____

Revision: How many ounces of carbonated beverages, such as Coca-Cola, Pepsi-Cola, ginger ale, or Sprite, did you drink today? _____

3. Don't write items that are ambiguous. Even common words that seem self-explanatory may have different meanings for people. Consider the word *family* in the following item. Does *family* include only members living in the household, the traditional nuclear family, all relatives, or people one lives with regardless of relationship? In the revision, the researcher first establishes that the participant lives with a family member, and then asks about that person's reliability for taking the participant to the doctor.

Weak: Can you count on a member of your family to take you to the doctor each week?

Yes_____ No_____

Revision: Do you live with a spouse, partner, adult children, or other adults?

Yes_____ No_____

If yes, can you count on one of them to take you to the doctor each week?

Yes_____ No_____

4. Don't write items that contain value-laden or biased words. Using terms that are emotionally or politically loaded will influence responses according to the perspective they establish. The word *proabortion* establishes a perspective different from that of the term *prochoice*. Likewise, the term *pro-life* establishes a perspective different from that of the term *antiabortion*.

Weak: Do you agree with the antienvironmentalist decision to cut down trees for the new school of the arts?

Yes_____ No_____

Revision: Do you agree with the administration's decision to cut down trees to build the new school of the arts?

Yes_____ No_____

Survey Format

When researchers are developing a survey, they need to make decisions about the order of the items and the manner of presentation. For printed surveys that participants will complete, the researcher must consider the cover page, the instructions, the font size, and the spacing of items. Dillman (2000) has written extensively about the tailored design method (TDM) of survey development. Although the focus of the TDM is on mail, telephone, and Internet surveys, we can apply some of its principles to any type of survey. Here, we present a brief overview of some of the key elements of a good survey.

Dillman (2000) recommends that the cover of a survey include a logo or other representation of the topic under consideration. For instance, a survey on health behaviors for adults might show men and women exercising. To save paper, some researchers put information about the study, including the necessary elements of informed consent, on the front cover. Dillman (2000) frowns on this choice, suggesting instead that information about the study and about informed consent be provided in a letter included with the survey.

When making decisions about the order of items, the researcher should begin with items that are related to the theme of the survey. If a survey is about motorcycle use, the first questions should query respondents about their use of motorcycles. Some researchers begin surveys by asking for background information such as age, education, race, and marital status. Although these questions are important, they should be placed at the end of the survey rather than at the beginning. People who are asked to complete a survey on motorcycle use and then are immediately asked their age will wonder about the intentions of the researcher. Another general principle is to place sensitive items, such as those asking about sex or illegal behaviors, around the midpoint of the survey or toward the end.

In considering the order of items on a survey, Clark and Schober (1992) note some interesting findings from their studies. First, people tend to use their earlier answers as evidence for later judgments. In other words, respondents feel pressure to be consistent in their responses throughout the survey. After they express an opinion, their responses to later questions will correspond to that opinion. If a person is unable to name the governor of Georgia at first, that person most likely will fail to express a great deal of interest in state government. The respondent is more likely to express little or no interest in state government. However, if the question about interest in state government appears first, the responses are likely to be more positive—that is, more people will express moderate or great interest in state government.

Second, people tend to interpret successive questions as related to the same topic unless they are told otherwise. Consider these two successive items from a chart review:

1. Was the person diagnosed with AIDS?
2. Was the diagnosis recorded on the chart?

In this example, is the researcher interested only in the diagnosis of AIDS being recorded on the chart? What if the person did not have AIDS? Does the researcher want to know whether other diagnoses are recorded as well? Given the sequence of the two items, the respondent might believe the researcher cares only about the diagnosis of AIDS and might fail to consider other diagnoses.

Third, when a general question follows a specific question on the same topic, an exclusive interpretation or an inclusive one may result, depending on the circumstances. For example, if a specific question that is asked first requests some information contained in the more general question that is asked second, the respondent is likely to exclude the information presented in the specific item when answering the more general question.

If a person is first asked, "How is your back today?" and then asked, "How are you feeling today?" that person is likely to first describe how his or her back is and then, in responding to the more general item about how he or she is feeling, exclude information about his or her back. Here, people may assume that they have already provided enough information about their backs, and that the questioner is interested in other aspects of their health.

Conversely, an item that is asked first may establish a perspective from which a respondent then chooses to answer a more general item. College students who are first asked to evaluate how happy they are with their dating may consider their response to this item when they are later asked to evaluate a more general item such as how happy they are with life in general (Strack, Martin, et al., 1988).

Many researchers place all the instructions for completing a survey on the first page. However, some people fail to begin a survey on the first page. They may complete items about which they are most knowledgeable or with which they are most comfortable and then move in a seemingly random way through the survey. To assist these individuals as well as those who begin at the beginning, the researchers should place instructions where they are needed. Instructions should occur before every transition in the type of item or the type of information requested. If respondents are required to skip some items based on their response to a particular item (in what are called *skip patterns*), arrows should direct the respondent to the next item that is appropriate to his or her response.

Regarding other aspects of the survey, the font size should take the respondents into consideration. Older individuals, in general, will appreciate a larger type size. Today, with computer technology, the researcher has a choice of fonts to enliven the survey. However, the cliché holds true: too much of a good thing could detract from the survey itself. Though researchers may choose unusual fonts for headings, they should stick to traditional fonts, such as Times Roman or Arial, for the items themselves. The researcher should also consider the spacing of items, allowing enough space between items to avoid crowding and illegibility. The respondent must be able to see clearly where to put the response for each item. Crowding items tends to increase respondent error.

Dillman (2000) suggests putting the survey in booklet form, with the front cover showing the logo and the back cover left blank. The researcher should use the last page to ask respondents about their experience with the survey.

Survey Administration

We can administer surveys in a variety of ways. Until near the end of the twentieth century, the most common methods of administration were face-to-face structured interviews and pencil-and-paper forms completed by participants. Computers have significantly changed the ways in which surveys are administered. Today, investigators may send surveys to participants by e-mail, or participants can log into a Web site to complete a survey. Hand-held and laptop computers allow direct entry of data into the computer database by the interviewer or the participant. Each approach has its own advantages and disadvantages, of which only a few will be discussed here.

In a face-to-face interview, the interviewer and the participant are physically together. The interviewer asks the questions and records the participant's answers. When using this format, the researcher must provide the interviewer with extensive training about the research study, the items themselves, and the proper manner of asking questions. The researcher also must decide which items should include probes for the interviewer to clarify information and must decide on the types of probes. The advantages of this approach include the likelihood that all items will be completed or that an explanation will be given for those items that are left unanswered. A probe might clarify items that are confusing to the participant, leading to more accurate answers. The disadvantages include a greater possibility of socially desirable responses because the participant must provide the answers to another human being. Also, the cost of the interviewer-administered survey is generally greater than the costs associated with other methods.

A second form of interviewer-administered survey is the telephone survey. In this approach, interviewers call the participant on the phone and read aloud items to which the participant responds. In addition to providing the opportunity to use probes and to clarify questions, the telephone interview is generally more convenient for both the interviewer and the participant because it does not require travel and it is generally shorter than other interviews. However, a distinct disadvantage is the inability of the participant to see the interviewer or the response options. In the face-to-face interview, the interviewer and respondent can see each other and use the full range of verbal and nonverbal cues in their discourse. In telephone interviews, where interviewer and respondent are unable to see each other, pauses are more disruptive and pressure to respond quickly increases. This means that the accuracy of responses in which recall and calculation are required is diminished. Because the respondent cannot see the response options, response choices to questions are limited to what people can reasonably remember and consider without a printed reminder.

In the third type of survey, respondents read and answer each item on their own. The traditional approach involves the use of paper and pencil to complete the survey. The survey instrument can be provided to the participants in a number of ways. Surveys can be handed out to individuals or sent by surface mail or email. Surveys can also be administered to large preformed groups, such as classes of students or attendees at a conference. Giving the survey to members of large groups has the advantage of collecting information from many participants at the same time. Generally, the paper-and-pencil survey is less costly than the face-to-face and telephone surveys. Whether administered individually or to a group, the paper-and-pencil survey allows respondents to answer the questions on their own at their own pace. On the negative side, the respondents must figure out for themselves the meanings of terms and how to complete the survey. Respondents sometimes fail to follow directions, fail to complete the items in the order presented, or make careless errors that decrease the quality of the data. Surveys administered to large preformed groups suffer from the lack of random sampling, which limits the generalizability of the results. Mail surveys are expensive, and researchers must make efforts to follow up with respondents who have failed to return surveys.

As we have mentioned, an increasingly popular approach for the administration of surveys is asking participants to record their answers directly into the computer. This approach has several advantages, including the elimination of the need for a data-entry person to enter responses from paper forms into the computer. Using computers with an audio component, each participant hears the same voice reading the same instructions. This feature enhances the consistency of survey administration and reduces measurement error related to misreading an item or related to the tone and accent of an interviewer's voice. When using the computer, participants are required to answer the items in the order presented, eliminating the possibility of missing items. Items that should be skipped based on previous responses are never shown to the respondent, thus reducing error associated with inconsistent responses. Recent studies also show that respondents are more likely to admit to sensitive behaviors such as drug use when using the computer as compared to participating in face-to-face interviews (Jones, 2003; Metzger, 2000). The primary disadvantages of using computers to administer surveys are related to the computer literacy of the staff and participants and to software glitches. Training staff and providing some initial assistance to participants are usually sufficient to overcome computer literacy issues. Software glitches, however, can result in the loss of one or more completed surveys. Procedures for monitoring and data transfer can help prevent major problems with data collection.

Summary

In this chapter, we have presented a brief description of the procedures of survey development and administration. An effective survey begins with a statement of purpose and a list of objectives. The objectives are used to determine the content of the survey and to guide the development of individual items. A major emphasis in this chapter was on item construction. The principles for writing high-quality items will be useful to the student when we discuss scale development in Chapter Seven. Students who are interested in more extensive discussion of survey development and administration will find the texts by Dillman (2000), Mangione (1995), Salant and Dillman (1994), and Schonlau, Fricker, and Elliott (2002) helpful. Likewise, those who are interested in more detailed discussion of issues related to item writing should read the classic text by Sudman and Bradburn (1982) and the more recent work by Sudman, Bradburn, and Schwarz (1996), Schwarz and Sudman (1996), and Tourangeau, Rips, and Rasinski (2000).

CHAPTER FIVE

KNOWLEDGE TESTS

LEARNING OBJECTIVES

At the end of this chapter, the student should be able to

1. Describe the characteristics of a knowledge test.
2. Discuss the basic principles of knowledge test construction.
3. Develop a table of test specifications.
4. Apply principles to writing multiple-choice and true/false items.
5. Revise poorly written items.
6. Describe the association between item wording and measurement error.
7. Conduct three types of item analyses.

There is a saying in health behavior research that knowledge does not predict behavior. For example, smokers are likely to know they are at risk for lung cancer, yet their knowledge of the risk seems to have little effect on their decision to smoke. Similarly, sunbathers are likely to understand the relationship between sun exposure and skin cancer risk. Still, many choose to spend hours in the sun without applying sunscreen. Despite the absence of a consistent association between knowledge and health behaviors, behavioral scientists occasionally want to find out what people know about health behavior. Take, for instance, a researcher studying hand-washing practices of medical residents. This researcher may want to consider what the residents know and do not know about infectious diseases and the correct hand-washing procedures. Or a health educator who offers an Internet-based diabetes self-management course may want to assess how much participants have learned about diabetes on completion of the program.

Behavioral scientists generally measure knowledge using simple tests. The development and evaluation of these tests receive little attention in the health behavior literature. As a result, behavioral scientists tend to use informal methods to create tests. A common approach to test construction is to review information sources in order to select content for a test, and then to reshape the content into test items. Often little attention is given to the primary use of the test and the quality of the items. Poorly constructed tests resulting from this process can produce misleading findings.

There is a significant body of literature on test construction and evaluation. However, this literature focuses primarily on achievement tests. Behavioral scientists who seek to develop high-quality knowledge tests must expend considerable effort to read this literature and determine the principles and procedures that are important in the development and evaluation of knowledge tests for behavioral research and health education. In this chapter, we present a brief introduction to some of the principles and practices that are useful to behavioral researchers and health educators in the development and evaluation of knowledge tests. We limit the discussion to the development and assessment of tests of knowledge of health information. This chapter presents the procedures for test construction, including stating the purpose, writing objectives, using a table of test specifications, and writing items. The discussion of writing items is limited to multiple-choice and true/false items, because these items are most likely to be used in health behavior research and evaluation. The discussion of test evaluation is limited to several simple procedures that health behavior researchers can use to assess the quality of items and the overall test.

Test Construction

Figure 5.1 presents the steps for test construction and evaluation. The five steps are (1) state the purpose of the test, (2) state the test objectives, (3) review content, (4) develop a table of test specifications, (5) write test items, and (6) conduct an item analysis to evaluate the quality of the items and that of the overall test.

State the Purpose of the Test

The test construction process begins with a statement of the purpose of the test. Among behavioral scientists, the three primary reasons for using knowledge tests are (1) to assess the knowledge base of a particular population on a particular health topic, (2) to determine whether knowledge of a health topic is related to behavior or attitudes

FIGURE 5.1. STEPS IN THE DEVELOPMENT OF A KNOWLEDGE TEST.

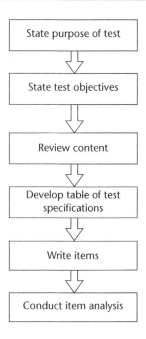

in a particular population, and (3) to determine whether knowledge of a health topic changes following an intervention. It is important to state the purpose of the test because the reason for measuring knowledge dictates to some extent the content, specificity, and difficulty level of the items included in the test. In the achievement test literature, the link between the purpose of the test and the characteristics of the test (type and difficulty of items) is fairly well established. It is generally accepted that there are two major uses of achievement tests (Gronlund, 1977). One is to rank students according to their test performance. This type of test, called a norm-referenced test, allows teachers to compare each student's performance with that of other students. The second type of test, called a criterion-referenced test, gauges the student's performance against preset criteria. In this type of test, the teacher is interested in the extent to which each student has met the objectives for the course. Unfortunately, the link between the primary uses of knowledge tests in health behavior research and the characteristics of the tests has not been fully addressed. However, drawing from the achievement test literature, we will provide some suggestions for the behavioral scientist and the health educator to consider when developing knowledge tests.

In addition to providing direction for the ultimate use of the test, the statement of purpose also places boundaries around the content to be tested. Suppose a researcher wants to find out how much college students know about HIV. Because HIV knowledge assessment could include many aspects—incidence, prevalence, transmission, prevention, treatment, antiretroviral medications, quality of life, access to care, current research, or cost—the researcher must decide which information is most important to collect from college students. Most students are unlikely to be knowledgeable about HIV treatments, research, costs, and access to care. Because college students are sexually active and many do not use condoms, the researcher's focus is most likely to be the students' knowledge of HIV transmission and prevention practices.

State the Test Objectives

After determining the general purpose of the test, the researcher lists specific objectives to guide the development of actual test items. The process of developing a test is much easier when specific test objectives are stated. In the achievement test literature, test objectives are synonymous with learning objectives. Learning objectives are developed for each course, and generally these objectives are used to create tests of the course content. There are several approaches to the development of learning objectives (Gronlund, 1978; Osterlind, 1998). One of the most common, the taxonomy of educational objectives, was developed by Bloom (1956). Bloom describes three primary domains of objectives: cognitive (knowledge), affective (attitudes or emotions), and psychomotor (skills). Because our focus is on knowledge tests, we present only the cognitive domain.

The six cognitive objectives from Bloom's taxonomy, in ascending order of complexity, are knowledge, comprehension, application, analysis, synthesis, and evaluation. Knowledge is the lowest level of complexity, requiring simple recall or recognition of information. Comprehension requires the translation of concepts or principles. Application is the use of concepts or principles in new situations. For example, defining the term *measurement* using one's own words demonstrates comprehension, and using rules for item writing demonstrates application. Analysis entails breaking down information. Synthesizing it means combining information to form a new product. Students who are asked to compare and contrast different approaches to scale development use analytic skills, and those who are asked to construct a scale use synthesis skills. Evaluation, at the highest level of complexity, involves appraisal of information. For example, the psychometric assessment of a scale designed to measure quality of life for use among women with breast cancer demonstrates the ability to evaluate information.

Bloom (1956) provides a list of verbs to develop learning objectives for each level of the cognitive objectives presented above. For knowledge, Bloom suggests using verbs such as *define, identify, list, know, name,* and *state.* A few objectives for a test of HIV knowledge might be:

• Define HIV.
• List three ways in which HIV can be transmitted.

- Name four strategies to prevent HIV.
- Identify five ways in which HIV cannot be transmitted.
- Identify five strategies that are ineffective in preventing HIV.
- Know that HIV cannot be cured.

In educational institutions, instructors use Bloom's cognitive objectives to develop learning objectives for courses. Teachers decide which information to present and test at each of the six levels. In fact, we developed the learning objectives at the beginning of each chapter in this book using Bloom's taxonomy. Health educators who develop and offer programs on health topics are likely to use a similar taxonomy to create program objectives. Likewise, behavioral scientists testing interventions to change behaviors are likely to state intervention objectives that indicate expected outcomes associated with participation in the interventions. In each case, learning objectives written to assess the cognitive domain (knowledge) can be used to create test objectives.

The situation for a researcher who wants to add a test of knowledge to a survey or who wants to examine the relationship between knowledge and a specific health behavior is a bit different. Generally, the researcher does not have a set of learning objectives from which to create test objectives. Instead, the researcher needs to consider carefully the content of the test and the population for which it is being developed. Using this information, the researcher can create a set of test objectives.

Review Content

After making a decision about the scope of the test, the researcher uses certain resources to obtain accurate information about the topic. These resources include a review of the literature, discussions with scientists or other experts in the topic area, and contact with agencies or organizations that provide information on the topic. For example, the Centers for Disease Control and Prevention (CDC) houses the most up-to-date information on HIV prevention. Our researcher who wants to test students' knowledge about HIV prevention would be wise to obtain literature from the CDC and visit the CDC Web site. In Chapter Seven, we will provide a more detailed discussion of the types of resources that can be used to develop test items.

Develop a Table of Test Specifications

Because behavioral scientists and health educators generally limit their assessment of the cognitive domain to that of knowledge, that is, the recall or recognition of facts, rules, or other information, we will emphasize tests of knowledge in the discussion that follows.

After the decision on the scope of the test and the review of materials, the researcher is ready to write the knowledge items. The item-writing process for tests begins with the development of a table of test specifications (also called a test blueprint). The table of specifications is a matrix in which the rows identify the content to be tested and the columns indicate the dimensions of that content. For educational tests, developers use cognitive objectives such as Bloom's as the test dimensions (columns).

Table 5.1 is a sample table of test specifications for a test for a course on measurement. The content domains are a definition of measurement, the history of measurement, types of questionnaire items, types of scales, and the item-writing process. This sample table of test specifications represents all six cognitive objectives—knowledge, comprehension, application, analysis, synthesis, and evaluation—in the columns. X's indicate the cognitive objective that will be assessed on the test for each content domain. For example, items written about the definition of measurement will be written at the knowledge level, whereas those written to assess the history of measurement will be written at both the knowledge and comprehension levels. Some items assessing the content of types of questionnaire items and scales will be written at the higher levels, including analysis, synthesis, and evaluation.

Table 5.2 is a more useful table of test specifications for test development. In this table, specific learning objectives make up the content domain (rows), and the cognitive objectives make up the dimensions (columns). Notice that rather than X's, there are numbers in the boxes, to indicate the number of items that will be written for each intersection of content and dimension.

A table of test specifications for a ten-item HIV knowledge test might look like Table 5.3. According to this table, the researcher will create a ten-item test with the following items: two items to measure knowledge of ways in which HIV can be transmitted, two for knowledge of ways in which it cannot be transmitted, two for knowledge of strategies that are effective in preventing HIV, two for knowledge of strategies that are ineffective, and one item each to measure knowledge about what HIV is and its ultimate outcome. The researcher will assess each item at the lowest level of cognitive complexity—knowledge.

Domain-Sampling Model

Notice that in Table 5.3, the researcher expects to write fewer items than those listed in the test objectives (presented earlier under test objectives). Although students may be expected to know many specific facts about HIV, the researcher anticipates that in his or her study the students will have only a few minutes to respond about their HIV knowledge. Thus, the investigator must make a decision about which items to include on the test. Sometimes researchers are concerned that a brief test may inadequately reflect students' knowledge. However, if the researcher develops and evaluates the test from a domain-sampling model perspective, ten items may prove sufficient to provide a reasonable estimate of the student's knowledge of HIV prevention. The

TABLE 5.1. SAMPLE TABLE OF TEST SPECIFICATIONS.

Content Domain	Cognitive Objectives					
	Knowledge	Comprehension	Application	Analysis	Synthesis	Evaluation
Definition of measurement	X					
History of measurement	X					
Types of questionnaire items	X	X	X	X	X	X
Types of scales	X	X	X	X	X	X
Item-writing process	X	X	X			X

TABLE 5.2. SAMPLE TABLE OF TEST SPECIFICATIONS USING INDIVIDUAL LEARNING OBJECTIVES.

Content Domain	Cognitive Objectives					
	Knowledge	Comprehension	Application	Analysis	Synthesis	Evaluation
Describe the characteristics of a survey		2				
Discuss the basic principles of survey construction		2				
Apply principles of item writing			2			
Revise poorly written items			2			
Describe the association between item wording and measurement error				2		

**TABLE 5.3. TABLE OF TEST SPECIFICATIONS FOR
AN HIV KNOWLEDGE TEST.**

Content Domain	Knowledge (# of Items)
List three ways in which HIV can be transmitted	2
Identify five ways in which HIV cannot be transmitted	2
Name four strategies to prevent HIV	2
Identify five strategies that are ineffective in preventing HIV	2
Define HIV	1
Know that HIV cannot be cured	1

domain-sampling model assumes that items selected for a test are a random sample of all possible items that measure the content of interest. We can develop a number of tests using a large pool of test items. Each test would be composed of a different set of items, but some items from one test might appear on another. If we select the items randomly, a student's scores on any one test will be strongly correlated with scores on all possible tests created from the same pool of items. Thus, any one test should provide a good estimate of the student's knowledge.

Figure 5.2 presents the domain-sampling model. The larger circle represents the pool of all possible items for a given content domain. The smaller circles represent randomly selected sets of items that make up individual tests. Each letter represents a test item. If randomization is conducted in such a way that items are replaced after selection for each test, an item can appear on more than one test.

FIGURE 5.2. DIAGRAM OF THE DOMAIN-SAMPLING METHOD.

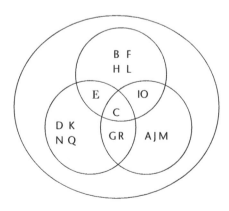

The domain-sampling method requires the development of a pool of items. The process of creating a large pool of items is time-consuming and sometimes impractical when a researcher plans to use just one knowledge test in a study. Even when not using the test pool, the researcher can develop more items than are required for the test. The researcher can then use the item analysis techniques presented later in this chapter to select the items that perform best for the population of interest.

Behavioral scientists often include all possible knowledge items in a given content domain to create a comprehensive test. For example, they may include all possible routes of HIV transmission on an HIV knowledge test. However, if the test is conceptualized within the domain-sampling model, scores on a test composed of an adequate representation of items should correlate with the scores on a test composed of a comprehensive set of items.

Types of Items

Multiple-choice and true/false items are the two primary types of items used on knowledge tests. In this section, we present criteria for constructing effective multiple-choice and true/false items. The multiple-choice item consists of a stem and a set of choices. The stem is the introductory statement for the multiple-choice item. For example, the question, "Which of the following is a way to prevent the spread of HIV?" is a stem and would be followed by three to five answer choices. Generally, only one of the answer choices is correct; the others function as distracters (plausible but incorrect responses). Respondents are instructed to select the answer choice that is the correct response or the best response. Responses are scored as correct or incorrect, and total scores are found by summing the number of correct responses. The number of correct responses can be converted to the percentage of correct responses by dividing the number of correct responses by the total number of items on the test and then multiplying by 100. A true/false item consists of a "statement of fact." The respondent evaluates the statement and determines whether it is true or false. Yes/no items are similar to true/false items in that they too require an evaluation of a statement. The statement, however, is presented in the form of a question to which the respondent answers yes or no. Correct responses for true/false and yes/no items are added to yield a total score. A percentage-correct score can also be computed for true/false and yes/no items.

Gronlund (1977) and Osterlind (1998) published basic guidelines for writing multiple-choice and true/false items. We rely on their work in presenting the guidelines that follow, first for multiple-choice items and then for true/false items. We use the guidelines to create an HIV knowledge test as an example.

Multiple-Choice Items

1. *Measure relevant information.* One of the first recommendations is the assessment of relevant information for a given population. If our researcher wants to develop a test to measure the HIV knowledge of college students, the information should be relevant to college students. A specialist in HIV may be able to answer an item related to the number of infants infected with HIV. However, because this information is unlikely to be of interest to or known by college students, a better item may ask instead about HIV transmission, which college students need to know about.

> *Low-relevance stem:* Overall, how many infants have been infected with HIV from their mothers since the beginning of the AIDS epidemic?
>
> *High-relevance stem:* HIV can be transmitted though which of the following routes?

2. *State a single, clear problem in the stem.* In the poor stem that follows, the introduction of both beliefs and myths can be confusing for respondents. The better stem is simple and to the point.

> *Poor stem:* People have many beliefs about how HIV is transmitted between persons. Some of these beliefs are correct and others are myths. Which of the following do you think is not a myth?
>
> *Better stem:* Which of the following events can lead to the transmission of HIV?

3. *State the stem in simple, clear language.* The following poor stem is convoluted and difficult to read, whereas the better stem is clearly stated.

> *Poor stem:* A reduction in HIV can be achieved by which of the following strategies designed to reduce transmission?
>
> *Better stem:* Which of the following can reduce the transmission of HIV?

4. *Put as much of the necessary wording as possible in the stem (don't repeat it in the answers).*

> *Poor stem:* Which of the following statements is not true?
> A. Birth control pills will not prevent HIV transmission.
> B. Urination after intercourse will not prevent HIV transmission.
> C. Condoms will not prevent HIV transmission.
> D. Cleaning needles with soap and water will not prevent HIV transmission.

Better stem: Which of the following can prevent transmission of HIV?

    A. Birth control pills
    B. Urination after intercourse
    C. Condoms
    D. Cleaning needles with soap and water

5. State the item in positive form.

Poor stem: Which of the following is not an effective HIV prevention strategy?

Better stem: Which of the following is an effective HIV prevention strategy?

6. Emphasize a negative word if it appears in the stem. Sometimes it is impossible to write a stem without using a negative word. In these cases, highlight the negative word to draw attention to it. Doing so will reduce errors due to misreading the stem.

Poor stem: HIV cannot be transmitted by . . .

Better stem: HIV *cannot* be transmitted by . . .

7. Make certain that the intended answer is the correct answer or the best answer. In the example of poor answer choices that follows, both cleaning needles and using condoms can be correct answers. In the item with better answer choices, only *condoms* is the correct answer.

Poor answer choices: Which of the following will prevent the transmission of HIV?

    A. Birth control pills
    B. Urination after intercourse
    C. Condoms
    D. Cleaning needles

Better answer choices: Which of the following will prevent the transmission of HIV?

    A. Birth control pills
    B. Urination after intercourse
    C. Condoms
    D. Cleaning needles with water

8. Make all answers grammatically consistent with the stem.

Poor answer choices: HIV is _____.

    A. a virus
    B. a bacterium
    C. has characteristics of both a virus and a bacterium
    D. no one really knows

Better answer choices: HIV is _____.

    A. a virus
    B. a bacterium
    C. a combination of a virus and a bacterium
    D. an unknown organism

9. Avoid verbal clues that lead to the correct answers or help eliminate incorrect answers. The poor stem that follows provides a clue that HIV is a virus.

Poor stem: Human immunodeficiency virus (HIV) is _____.

    A. a virus
    B. a bacterium
    C. a combination of a virus and a bacterium
    D. an unknown organism

Better stem: HIV is _____.

10. Make distracters plausible and appealing. In the following example of poor answer choices, one of the distracters (incorrect responses) is *reading about HIV.* Most college students would immediately identify this choice as incorrect or implausible. Likewise, wearing a copper bracelet has not been associated with HIV prevention and may not function as a plausible distracter. In the better answer choices, the distracters of washing one's hands, using birth control pills, and cleaning needles with water are likely to be more plausible because both washing of hands and cleaning of needles are activities generally engaged in to prevent infection. Some students believe that birth control pills will prevent sexually transmitted diseases as well as pregnancy.

Poor answer choices: Sexually active people can reduce their risk of contracting HIV by

    A. wearing a copper bracelet
    B. using birth control pills
    C. using condoms
    D. reading about HIV

Better answer choices: Sexually active people can reduce their risk of contracting HIV by

    A. washing their hands
    B. using birth control pills
    C. using condoms
    D. cleaning needles with water

11. Use "All of the above" and "None of the above" as responses sparingly.

Poor answer choices: Which of the following is a way to transmit HIV?

    A. Unprotected sex
    B. Unclean needles
    C. HIV-infected mother to infant
    D. All of the above

Better answer choices: Which of the following lists the three primary ways of transmitting HIV?

    A. Unprotected sex, unclean needles, HIV-infected mother to infant
    B. Unprotected sex, unclean kitchen utensils, mosquitoes
    C. Unprotected sex, unclean needles, mosquitoes
    D. Unprotected sex, unclean kitchen utensils, HIV-infected mother to infant

12. Use the two-layered response option sparingly.
The two-layered item consists of two sets of options. The first set consists of all correct, all incorrect, or a combination of correct and incorrect answer choices. The second set of options contains combinations of the answer choices presented in the first set of options. The task for the respondent is to select the correct response from the second set of options. Because it requires two judgments, the two-layered item is more complex than the typical multiple-choice item. As shown here, presenting just the second set of options with an appropriate stem simplifies the item.

Poor answer choices: Which of the following is a way to transmit HIV?

1. Unprotected sex
2. Kissing
3. HIV-infected mother to infant
4. Mosquitoes

A. 1 and 2 only
B. 1 and 3 only
C. 1, 2, and 3
D. 1, 3, and 4

Better answer choices: Which of the following lists the three primary ways of transmitting HIV?

A. Unprotected sex, unclean needles, HIV-infected mother to infant
B. Unprotected sex, unclean kitchen utensils, mosquitoes
C. Unprotected sex, unclean needles, mosquitoes
D. Unprotected sex, unclean kitchen utensils, HIV-infected mother to infant

13. *Make each item independent.* If the answers to two items are interdependent, the respondent who selects the wrong answer for the first item has a high probability of selecting the wrong answer for the second item. A fairer test is produced by making the items independent.

1. Which of the following lists the three primary ways of transmitting HIV?

A. Unprotected sex, unclean needles, HIV-infected mother to infant
B. Unprotected sex, unclean kitchen utensils, mosquitoes
C. Unprotected sex, unclean needles, mosquitoes
D. Unprotected sex, unclean kitchen utensils, HIV-infected mother to infant

2. For which of the three primary modes of transmission mentioned above can medications be used to reduce the likelihood of transmission?

A. Unprotected sex
B. Mosquitoes
C. Needles or utensils
D. HIV-infected mother to infant

The correct answer for the first question is A, and the correct answer for the second question is D (HIV-infected mother to infant). If a respondent selected B or C to answer question 1, there is a possibility that he or she would select B, the wrong answer, for question 2.

One way to unlink the two questions would be to change the stem for question 2 as follows: "For which of the following modes of transmission can drugs be used to reduce the likelihood of transmission?"

14. Vary the position of the correct answer in a random fashion. After developers complete the set of items, they review the positions of the correct answers. If the correct answer often falls in a certain position (for example, frequently answer C is correct), respondents may use this placement as a clue to select the correct answer. After test developers determine the order of the items, they should position the correct answers by random selection or a similar process to vary their positions.

15. Vary the length of the correct answer to eliminate length as a clue. Ideally, answer choices are of similar length. (Of course, this parity is sometimes impossible to achieve.) When the correct answer is always the longest or the shortest in a set of items, respondents will use this clue to select the correct answer. Thus, when reviewing items, make certain that the correct answer varies in length and is consistently neither the shortest nor the longest choice.

True/False Items

The following are recommendations for writing true/false and yes/no items.

1. Include only one central significant idea in each statement.

Poor: A person can get HIV from mosquitoes and toilet seats.
Better: A person can get HIV from mosquitoes.

2. Word the statement so precisely that respondents can judge it as unequivocally true or false. The poor item shown here does not contain the qualification that the partner has HIV. Thus, a respondent could reason that the statement is true only under certain conditions.

Poor: Can a person get HIV through having sexual intercourse?
Better: Can a person get HIV by having sexual intercourse with someone who is infected with HIV?

3. Keep the statements short and keep the language structure simple.

Poor: Human immunodeficiency virus is the same thing as acquired immuno-deficiency syndrome.

Better: HIV is the same as AIDS.

4. Use negative statements sparingly.
Items containing negative words such as *not* and prefixes such as *un-* and *non-* are frequently misread by respondents. If a negative term is used, emphasize it.

Poor: A person cannot get HIV from mosquitoes.

Better: A person *cannot* get HIV from mosquitoes.

An even better approach is to eliminate the word *not* (this will also change the correct answer).

A person can get HIV from mosquitoes.

5. Avoid double negatives.

Poor: A person cannot reduce his or her chances of getting HIV by not shaking hands with someone who has HIV.

Better: A person can get HIV by shaking hands with someone who has HIV.

6. Attribute statements of opinion to some source.

Poor: People should use condoms to reduce their chances of contracting HIV.

Better: According to the CDC, sexually active people should use condoms to reduce their chances of contracting HIV.

7. Avoid extraneous clues to the answer.

Poor: Condoms help prevent HIV; therefore, people can reduce their chance of getting HIV by using a condom when they have sexual intercourse.

Better: People can reduce their chance of getting HIV by using a condom when they have sexual intercourse.

8. Randomly vary the sequence of true statements and false statements (or yes statements and no statements). After completing the set of items, review it for percentages of true statements and of false statements. Ideally, half of the items will be true and half will be false. Developers should order the items randomly to prevent a pattern of true and false statements that could serve as a clue for respondents.

Item Analysis

After creating a knowledge test, the developers should examine the test to identify poor items. The assessment is conducted to evaluate each item and the total test with the goal of creating a test that will adequately reflect the knowledge of the people who answer the items. The researcher can use several simple procedures, broadly defined as item analysis, to evaluate individual items as well as the total test. We will discuss three of these methods: item-objective congruency, difficulty index, and discrimination index. The first uses content specialists who evaluate the extent to which each item measures the content that the test is intended to measure. The second assesses the difficulty level of each item, and the third gives an assessment of how well the items discriminate among groups of participants. Researchers can use information from each of these assessments to improve individual items as well as the test as a whole.

Item-Objective Congruency

Sometimes called the judgmental approach (Osterlind, 1998), the item-objective congruency method uses content experts. The experts selected to conduct the assessment of the test should be individuals with expertise in the content area. Thus, for the HIV knowledge test, our experts might include scientists studying HIV, CDC staff in the HIV division, public health professionals involved in HIV prevention projects, and clinicians who care for people infected with HIV.

We first ask the experts to review the content and structure of each test item and of the total test. In this process, the experts read each item and its intended answer and evaluate these components for correctness and completeness. The most important aspect of this task is to determine whether each item is accurate and the answer correct based on current understanding in the field. The experts also evaluate the grammar and suggest wording changes to improve the items. Finally, the experts evaluate the set of items as a whole. In doing so, they assess the extent to which the test items adequately represent the content selected for inclusion in the test. In this global assessment, the experts can identify items for deletion as well as suggest additional items or content for inclusion.

Following the global assessment, the experts evaluate the extent to which the items correspond to the test objectives written by the test developer. To conduct this assessment, we give the experts the list of test objectives that were used to write the test items. The experts read each item and then rate each item on every objective. Osterlind (1998) suggests assigning −1 for an item that is a poor match with an objective, 0 for a moderate or uncertain match, and +1 for a strong match.

The ratings from all the experts are reviewed for correspondence with the intended objective and for agreement among the experts. Each item for which a majority of experts agree that it corresponds to its intended objective is retained. Each item that a majority of experts fail to link with its intended objective is either revised or eliminated, as is each item for which the experts show significant disagreement about its intended objective. Hambleton, Swaminathan, Algina, and Coulsen (1978) suggest that for an item to be retained, the number of experts who agree should be equal to $n - 1$. Thus, if there are four experts, three of them $(n - 1)$ must give a rating of +1 to the intended objective for an item to be retained. A rough estimate of the item-objective congruency for three out of four agreements is .75. For reviews by six experts, five experts would be required to agree, yielding a rough item-objective congruency estimate of .83. The following example will help illuminate this process.

Exhibits 5.1 and 5.2 present an example of materials that would be given to content experts to complete the task of evaluating item-objective congruency. The materials include (1) an instruction sheet describing the procedures for the evaluation, (2) a description of the instrument, including its intended uses, (3) the test objectives, (4) the test items, and (5) a rating sheet. The task for the content experts is first to evaluate the content and structure of each item and, second, to rate each item for objective congruency using the −1 to +1 rating scale.

Table 5.4 presents the results of an item-objective congruency evaluation conducted by three content experts for the ten-item HIV Knowledge Test. The rating for each expert is recorded in each of the cells of the matrix. Notice that all the experts gave a rating of +1 to each of the intended objectives (marked with an asterisk). However, for the majority of the items, one or more of the experts also indicated that the item could measure a second or third objective. For these items, the test developer can use comments on the rating forms or interviews with the experts to determine the reasons for their ratings. Information gained from these sources can be used to retain these items as is or modify them as necessary. It should be noted that items sometimes do measure more than one objective (Turner & Carlson, 2003). Thus, items would not necessarily be eliminated because experts failed to agree on only one objective.

The estimate of item-objective congruency for each of the ten items is 1.0, meaning that all three experts agreed on the intended objective for each of the items. The calculation of this estimate considers only the ratings in the cell of the intended

EXHIBIT 5.1. MATERIALS FOR REVIEW OF KNOWLEDGE ITEMS BY CONTENT EXPERTS.

Thank you for agreeing to review and evaluate the HIV knowledge test we have developed for our study of HIV prevention practices among college students. You were selected for this task because of your interest and expertise in HIV prevention and the development of knowledge tests used to measure HIV knowledge.

At this time, we need your assistance in assessing the congruency between the items we developed and the objectives that guided the development of the items. This task involves rating the congruency of each item with each objective.

The following information is included:

1. Description of the framework for test development
2. Description of the test
3. Test objectives
4. Test items
5. Form for rating item-objective congruency

The procedure for this task is

1. Read the description of the HIV knowledge test.
2. Read each item and its answer and determine the accuracy and completeness of the information.
3. Using the rating form, rate each item as to the degree of congruency between it and each objective using a +1, 0, −1 rating scale.
4. On the form itself, make any suggestions for the addition or deletion of items or changes in the wording of items.
5. Evaluate the instructions for the scale.
6. Evaluate the format of the scale.

DESCRIPTION OF THE HIV KNOWLEDGE TEST

The HIV Knowledge Test is a ten-item test designed to measure knowledge of HIV transmission and prevention practices. We used Bloom's taxonomy as the framework for developing the six test objectives on which the test is based. Each test objective is stated at the knowledge level of Bloom's taxonomy. That is, the test objectives are related to recall or recognition of facts or information. The six test objectives are

- Define HIV.
- List three ways in which HIV can be transmitted.
- Name four strategies to prevent HIV.
- Identify five ways in which HIV cannot be transmitted.
- Identify five strategies that are ineffective in preventing HIV.
- Know that HIV cannot be cured.

We used these six objectives to guide the development of our ten test items. We developed the test to assess the knowledge that college students possess related to HIV and AIDS. Once developed and evaluated, the test will be used in research studies to assess the HIV knowledge of college students. This test is composed of ten statements about HIV. Each statement is evaluated and rated as true or false. Correct responses to each item are summed to yield a total score. Total scores range from 0 to 10; higher scores indicate more knowledge about HIV.

HIV KNOWLEDGE TEST FOR COLLEGE STUDENTS

Directions: Below are ten statements about HIV. Please circle T if you think the statement is true or F if you think the statement is false.

	True	**False**
1. A person can reduce his or her chances of contracting HIV by having only one sexual partner.	**T**	F
2. Birth control pills help prevent the spread of HIV.	T	**F**
3. A person can get HIV by kissing a person infected with HIV.	T	**F**
4. HIV can be cured if treated early.	T	**F**
5. A person can get HIV by having unprotected sex with a person infected with HIV.	**T**	F
6. A person can get HIV by using unclean needles.	**T**	F
7. A person can get HIV from a mosquito bite.	T	**F**
8. A person can reduce his or her chances of contracting HIV by not having sexual intercourse with anyone.	**T**	F
9. Lambskin condoms help prevent the spread of HIV.	T	**F**
10. HIV is a virus.	**T**	F

Note: Correct answers shown here in boldface.

EXHIBIT 5.1. MATERIALS FOR REVIEW OF KNOWLEDGE ITEMS BY CONTENT EXPERTS (continued).

ITEM-OBJECTIVE CONGRUENCY RATING FORM

Instructions: On this form, please rate the extent to which each item corresponds with each objective. Six test objectives are listed in the columns and the ten items are listed in the rows. Please read the objective first and then the item. Rate each item on the three-point scale in terms of how closely it matches each objective. Because items were written for specific objectives, it is anticipated that items will not be perfect matches for each objective. Thus, consider the full range of the ratings below in evaluating each item-objective combination.

−1 = Item is a poor match with the objective
0 = Item is a moderate match with the objective or it is difficult to determine
+1 = Item is a strong match with the objective

	List three ways HIV can be transmitted.	List five ways HIV cannot be transmitted.	List four ways to prevent HIV.	Identify five strategies that are ineffective in preventing HIV.	Define HIV.	Know that HIV cannot be cured.
1. A person can reduce his or her chances of contracting HIV by having only one sexual partner.						
2. Birth control pills help prevent the spread of HIV.						
3. A person can get HIV by kissing a person infected with HIV.						
4. HIV can be cured if treated early.						
5. A person can get HIV by having unprotected sex with a person infected with HIV.						
6. A person can get HIV by using unclean needles.						
7. A person can get HIV from a mosquito bite.						
8. A person can reduce his or her chances of contracting HIV by not having sexual intercourse with anyone.						
9. Lambskin condoms help prevent the spread of HIV.						
10. HIV is a virus.						

TABLE 5.4. ITEM-OBJECTIVE CONGRUENCY EVALUATION CONDUCTED BY THREE CONTENT EXPERTS FOR TEN ITEMS.

	List three ways HIV can be transmitted.	List five ways HIV cannot be transmitted.	List four ways to prevent HIV.	Identify five strategies that are ineffective in preventing HIV.	Define HIV.	Know that HIV cannot be cured.
1. A person can reduce his or her chances of contracting HIV by having only one sexual partner.	+1 0 -1	-1 -1 -1	* +1 +1 +1	-1 -1 -1	-1 -1 -1	-1 -1 -1
2. Birth control pills help prevent the spread of HIV.	-1 -1 -1	-1 -1 -1	-1 -1 -1	* +1 +1 +1	-1 -1 -1	-1 -1 -1
3. A person can get HIV by kissing a person infected with HIV.	-1 0 -1	* +1 +1 +1	-1 -1 -1	-1 -1 -1	-1 -1 -1	-1 -1 -1
4. HIV can be cured if treated early.	-1 -1 -1	-1 -1 -1	-1 -1 -1	-1 -1 -1	-1 -1 -1	* +1 +1 +1
5. A person can get HIV by having unprotected sex with a person infected with HIV.	* +1 +1 +1	-1 -1 -1	+1 -1 -1	-1 -1 -1	-1 -1 -1	-1 -1 -1
6. A person can get HIV by using unclean needles.	* +1 +1 +1	0 -1 -1	0 -1 -1	-1 -1 -1	-1 -1 -1	-1 -1 -1
7. A person can get HIV from a mosquito bite.	-1 -1 -1	* +1 +1 +1	-1 -1 -1	-1 0 -1	-1 -1 -1	-1 -1 -1
8. A person can reduce his or her chances of contracting HIV by not having sexual intercourse with anyone.	-1 0 0	-1 -1 -1	* +1 +1 +1	-1 0 -1	-1 -1 -1	-1 -1 -1
9. Lambskin condoms help prevent the spread of HIV.	-1 -1 -1	-1 -1 -1	-1 0 -1	* +1 +1 +1	-1 -1 -1	-1 -1 -1
10. HIV is a virus.	-1 -1 -1	-1 -1 -1	-1 -1 -1	-1 -1 -1	* +1 +1 +1	-1 -1 -1

* Items that correspond to the objective.

objective for each item. Though this estimate can give the behavioral scientist or health educator a rough indication of the adequacy of each item, it is only an approximation of the item-objective congruency index. When a test will be used for evaluation of achievement, a more rigorous index of item-objective congruency is needed. This index takes into account all the experts' ratings in all the cells of the matrix. The calculation of the item-objective congruency index is complex and will not be presented here. However, the health educator or behavioral scientist who is interested in a more rigorous assessment of item-objective congruency is referred to the work of Hambleton, Swaminathan, Algina, and Coulson (1978), Crocker and Algina (1986), and Turner and Carlson (2003).

Average Congruency Percentage. The average congruency percentage provides an indication of how congruent the overall test is with the content domain (Popham, 1978). The average congruency percentage is calculated by first obtaining the percentage of items that each expert rated as +1, that is, congruent with its objective. The individual percentages of all the judges are summed and divided by the number of experts to obtain the average congruency percentage.

If five experts evaluated our HIV knowledge test and their percentages of items judged to be congruent were .90, .70, .80, .90, and .90, then the average congruency percentage would be 84. Average congruency percentages range from 0 percent to 100 percent. Waltz, Strickland, and Lenz (1991) suggest an average congruency percentage of at least .90 as acceptable. They also suggest including some items that are clearly wrong, to assess the attentiveness of experts in completing the task. Researchers might remove from the calculations the scores of experts who fail to notice the problematic items.

Difficulty Index

A second method of assessing knowledge items is the calculation of a difficulty index. The difficulty index and the discrimination index (described in the next section) require the collection of data from a sample of respondents. For this evaluation, the researcher should select individuals from the same population for which the knowledge test is being developed. Thus, the researcher who wants to test HIV knowledge among college students would select a sample of college students for the test. Ideally, the researcher has developed more items than are needed for the final version of the test. Information obtained from the participants will allow the researcher to select the best set of items for the knowledge test.

The difficulty index for dichotomous items is simply the proportion of people who answered an item correctly. It is also called the p value, and is not to be confused with the p value that denotes statistical significance. To calculate the difficulty index, we divide the number of people who answered the item correctly by the total number of participants as follows:

$$p = \frac{n_c}{N}$$

where

p = p value or difficulty index,
n_c = number of respondents who answered correctly, and
N = total number of respondents.

The difficulty index ranges in value from 0 (no one answers the item correctly) to 1.0 (everyone answers the item correctly). The difficulty index is interpreted to mean that the greater the proportion of test takers who answer the item correctly, the easier the item. Table 5.5 presents the p values and discrimination indexes for three items on a true/false HIV knowledge test. The p value for item 4 is .90 and that for item 9 is .68. For item 4, 90 percent of the respondents answered the item correctly, indicating that it was relatively easy for this group of participants to answer, whereas 68 percent of respondents answered item 9 correctly, suggesting that this item was more difficult to answer.

Researchers can also compute a difficulty index for both correct and incorrect responses on a multiple-choice test. This index is often adjusted to account for guessing (see Crocker & Algina, 1986). The researcher can compare the p values for the incorrect answer choices to determine which distracters are most appealing to respondents. Researchers should revise distracters that are seldom or never selected to make them more attractive options. Consider the p values of answer choices to the three multiple-choice items on HIV knowledge presented in Table 5.6. The correct answer for item 1 is C,

TABLE 5.5. EXAMPLE OF ITEM ANALYSIS FOR A TRUE/FALSE HIV KNOWLEDGE TEST.

	Difficulty Index p	Index of Discrimination $p - p^2 = D$
4. HIV can be cured if treated early.	.90	.90 − .81 = .09
7. A person can get HIV from a mosquito bite.	.77	.77 − .59 = .18
9. Lambskin condoms help prevent the spread of HIV.	.68	.68 − .46 = .22

which was selected by 90 percent of the respondents. Respondents did not select the incorrect answer choices A and D, and only 10 percent of them chose B. These results indicate that item 1 was especially easy for this group of respondents or that the distracters were unattractive alternatives. For item 2, answer choice B is correct; 50 percent of respondents selected this option. Answer choices C and D appear to be functioning as distracters, but answer choice A does not. Finally, the correct answer choice for item 3 was selected by only 30 percent of the respondents. However, answer choice D functioned as a powerful but incorrect alternative. Additional information from item discrimination, discussed later, will help the researcher decide whether to retain or revise item 3.

The p value tells the test developer how each item is performing (difficulty/ease). We can use the p value to compare the difficulty levels among a set of items for a given group of participants. For norm-referenced achievement tests, the range of p values for correct responses is .6 to .8, that is, between 60 percent and 80 percent of the respondents answer each item correctly (Crocker & Algina, 1986). In Table 5.6, item 2 meets this criterion, but items 1 and 3 do not. Because one goal of a knowledge test for course material is to make items neither too easy nor too difficult, a range of difficulty between .6 and .8 is ideal.

The researcher using a knowledge test as part of a research study may choose to use different p values depending on the use of the test. For example, the researcher may be interested in examining the overall HIV knowledge of college students rather than the achievement of any one student. Thus, the researcher may be content with higher-than-recommended p values. Nevertheless, the calculation of p values gives the researcher a gauge that indicates which items are easier or more difficult for participants. For multiple-choice tests, the p value also provides information about which distracters the respondents find most appealing.

TABLE 5.6. P VALUES FOR ANSWER CHOICES ON THREE MULTIPLE-CHOICE ITEMS ON AN HIV KNOWLEDGE TEST.

	Response Options			
Item	A	B	C	D
Item 1	0	.10	.90[a]	0
Item 2	0	.50[a]	.20	.30
Item 3	.30[a]	.20	.10	.40

[a] Correct response for the item.

Item Discrimination Index

A third method of assessing individual items is examination of the ability of the items to discriminate between test takers who know the content and those who do not know it well. Items that everyone answers correctly and items that no one answers correctly are useless in discerning differences in ability among test takers. Lord and Novick (1968, p. 329) proposed the following formula to compute an item discrimination index:

$$D = p - p^2$$

where

D = the item discrimination index,
p = the proportion of test takers who answer the item
      correctly (this is also the item difficulty estimate), and
p^2 = the square of p.

D is equivalent to the variance of the responses. The higher the variance, the more the item discriminates among the test takers. Using data from a sample of respondents, item discrimination indexes can be calculated for each item. These values can be used to select items that have high discrimination indexes. According to Lord and Novick (1968), items that have higher discrimination indexes contribute more to total test score variance. For multiple-choice and true/false (or yes/no) items, D is highest when $p = .5$. When p is near 0 or 1, an item cannot contribute to differentiation among test takers because the total score variance among test takers is low.

Table 5.5 presents the index of discrimination for three items on the HIV knowledge test. Notice that the values of D increase as the value of p approaches .5. Item 9, which has the highest difficulty index, also has the most discriminating power. The difficulty index is group-specific, meaning that one group of individuals might find items more difficult to answer than another group. For our HIV knowledge test, college freshmen might find the items relatively easy to answer, whereas eighth-grade students might experience more difficulty in answering the items.

Summary

Health professionals often have an interest in evaluating the knowledge of health behavior. This chapter has presented guidelines for developing simple tests of knowledge that are composed primarily of multiple-choice and true/false items. The test construction task is made much easier when the test developer begins by first stating a clear purpose and then writing learning objectives based on the content to be assessed. These learning objectives can be used to create a table of test specifications. This test matrix can in turn be used to ensure a representative sample of the content. This chapter has also presented three simple but useful ways of evaluating the adequacy of the test items: item-objective congruency, the difficulty index, and the discrimination index.

CHAPTER SIX

THEORY AND MEASUREMENT

LEARNING OBJECTIVES

At the end of this chapter, the student should be able to

1. Discuss the link between theory and measurement.
2. Draw the Gibbs model for selected concepts.
3. Diagram relationship statements using theory.
4. Differentiate between theoretical and operational definitions.
5. Describe the differences between surveys and scales.
6. State two advantages of multiple-item scales.
7. Give two reasons for developing a new health behavior scale.
8. Identify the purpose of a concept analysis.
9. Discuss techniques for conducting a concept analysis.
10. Identify the dimensions of a selected concept.
11. Identify the ways in which a selected concept is the same as or different from another concept.
12. Write a model case of a selected concept.

Matt, whom we met in Chapter One, is the project director of a recently funded study to evaluate the outcomes of a nutrition and exercise program for people over sixty-five. One of Matt's first assignments was to locate instruments that could be used to assess variables in the study. The study is based on social cognitive theory, and two concepts that will be assessed are self-efficacy and outcome expectations (OE). Matt has been able to locate scales to measure self-efficacy for healthy eating, self-efficacy for exercise, and OE for exercise to use among elderly people. However, he has not been able to find a scale to measure OE for healthy eating.

In order to have all the scales available to present at a team meeting, Matt and several other staff members met to construct a scale to measure the degree to which a person expects positive outcomes associated with healthy eating (OE for healthy eating). They began by reviewing the definition of the concept of OE. Then the staff members worked together to create items. When ten items had been written and agreed upon, the staff was satisfied that their task was complete.

Matt presented the scales at the next team meeting. The principal investigator was pleased that Matt and the staff had taken the initiative to meet the goal of obtaining scales to measure the study variables. Yet he expressed concern about the informal approach that the staff had used to develop the scale for OE for healthy eating. He wondered, for example, how the staff, all of whom were under thirty-five, knew that the items they had decided were important to assess were consistent with outcomes that might be selected by older men and women, many of whom suffer from chronic illness.

As we will see, the first line of defense against measurement error is the careful and thoughtful development of scales. Unfortunately, Matt and other researchers sometimes rush into scale development to meet a deadline for a project. Yet, as the principal investigator pointed out, a scale that receives little attention during the development phase may yield data that are useless for answering important research questions. In this chapter, we begin the study of scale development and evaluation. The entire process, which will be covered in the next seven chapters, is presented in Figure 6.1. This chapter focuses on the conceptualization process in scale development. It begins with a discussion of the link between theory and measurement. In this chapter, we will also learn concept analysis, an important precursor to the task of item writing.

Linking Measurement to Theory-Based Health Practice and Research

Health behavior and health education research often depend on the measurement of abstract constructs and concepts. In these cases, measurement must be extended to include the process of converting abstract concepts into empirical indicators—the actual methods or instruments used to measure the concepts. Empirical indicators can include

FIGURE 6.1. STEPS IN THE SCALE DEVELOPMENT PROCESS.

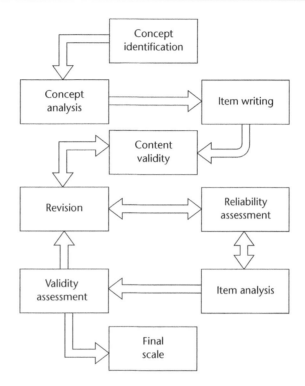

any of the instruments we presented in Chapter Two (for example, self-report questionnaires, observations, chart reviews, and physiological measures).

In behavioral research, scale development begins with a thorough understanding of the concept to be measured. The measurement process then proceeds to writing the items, stating the rules for using the scale, and devising scoring methods. The measurement process concludes with the assignment of a numeric score, generally corresponding to the type of conceptual dimensions or the amount (quantity) of the variable. We arrive at the numeric score through established rules and scoring methods. Figure 6.2 depicts the measurement process in health behavior research and evaluation. (As with any form of measurement, error is an undesirable but expected component.)

FIGURE 6.2. THE MEASUREMENT PROCESS IN HEALTH BEHAVIOR RESEARCH.

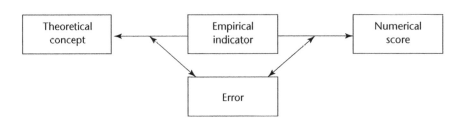

Gibbs's Model

As a student in public health, you have had some exposure to the predominant theories explaining health behavior, its antecedents, and its outcomes. These theories include:

- Health belief model (Rosenstock, 1960)
- Theory of planned behavior (Ajzen, 1991)
- Social cognitive theory (Bandura, 1997)
- Transtheoretical model (Prochaska & DiClemente, 1982)
- Diffusion of innovation (Rogers, 1995)
- Stress and coping theory (Lazarus & Folkman, 1984)

Each theory or model proposes a set of concepts (for example, perceived barriers and benefits, subjective norms, self-efficacy, OE, stress, and coping), and each proposes ways in which the concepts work together to determine or explain health behavior or other aspects of health. We refer to the associations among concepts proposed within the theory as relational statements (Gibbs, 1972). These associations are often depicted by using arrows to link related concepts. The arrow links the concept considered to be the cause (or the one that logically precedes the concept that follows it) to the concept considered to be the outcome (or the one that follows the first concept). For example, social cognitive theory (SCT) states that people who have higher levels of self-efficacy and more positive OE related to a particular behavior are more likely to engage in that behavior.

Behavioral theorists tend to use terms for concepts that fail to indicate exactly what quantity the concept measures (Mulaik, 2004). Thus an important next step is to state the concept as a variable in quantifiable terms. For example, if the self-efficacy

FIGURE 6.3. EXAMPLE OF RELATIONAL STATEMENTS IN SOCIAL COGNITIVE THEORY.

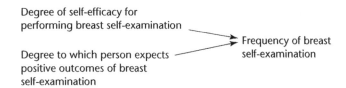

variable is "the degree to which one feels self-efficacious in performing a breast self-examination," OE might be "degree to which one expects positive outcomes from performing a breast self-examination," and breast self-examination might be "how often one performs a breast self-examination." Figure 6.3 depicts these relationships among variables. The two relational statements are

1. Women who report higher degrees of self-efficacy for performing breast self-examination will report more frequent breast self-examinations.
2. Women who report more positive OE related to performing breast self-examinations will report more frequent breast self-examinations.

If we want to test these theoretical associations, we must first understand and define the concepts—self-efficacy, outcome expectations, and breast self-examination. Then we must develop instruments to measure the concepts. The process whereby an investigator defines a concept in theoretical terms and then makes decisions as to how to measure it empirically is called a transformational statement (Gibbs, 1972). After researchers develop the instrument, they next devise rules to assign a numeric score that adequately reflects the amount of the concept possessed. Figure 6.4 illustrates the entire process, as proposed by Gibbs (1972), using terms later modified by Dulock and Holzemer (1991).

We give relational statements different names (that is, *axiom*, *proposition*, *theorem*, and *hypothesis*) at each level of the model depicting the relationship. As noted in the model, higher-level constructs might be transformed into lower-level concepts before the selection or development of measurement tools. Each concept must be transformed into an empirical indicator and stated as a variable in order to collect empirical data. Finally, a set of rules and procedures must be created in order to arrive at a numeric score that can be used in statistical analysis.

As shown in Figure 6.4, we can divide Gibbs's model into a conceptual component and an empirical component, and the transformational statement serves as a bridge be-

FIGURE 6.4. GIBBS'S RELATIONAL MODEL (1972) AS MODIFIED BY DULOCK AND HOLZEMER (1991).

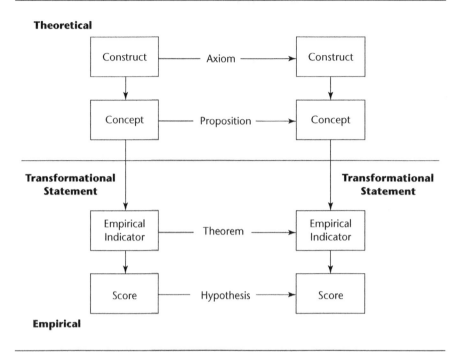

Source: Permission from J. Gibbs (2004).

tween the two components. Within the conceptual component, relationships between concepts are presented in abstract terms. For example, we might say that the concept of self-efficacy is associated with the health behavior of breast self-examination. The relational statement might be that women who report higher degrees of self-efficacy for performing a breast self-examination will report more frequent self-examinations. However, in the empirical part of the model, we are concerned with exactly how to measure each concept. Our concerns here are (1) the type of measuring instrument needed to measure the concepts and (2) how we will assign numeric scores using our measuring instruments. For our example, we might choose self-report measures in which we first ask women to rate, using a ten-point scale, how confident they are about performing a breast self-examination and then ask how often they performed the behavior in the past year. We then assign numeric scores to the responses, using predetermined rules. We use the numeric scores to perform statistical tests and the results of the statistical tests to determine whether a statistically significant positive correlation exists between the scores on the self-efficacy measure and the scores on the breast self-examination measure. If one does exist, we have evidence to support the theoretical statement that there is a positive relationship between the degree of self-efficacy to perform breast self-examinations and the frequency of breast self-examination.

Theoretical and Operational Definitions

As with everything in measurement, we must provide precise definitions of our concepts. Two terms important in the measurement process are *theoretical definitions* and *operational definitions*. A theoretical definition is one in which the meaning of the concept (or construct) is given by substituting other words or phrases for it (Waltz, Strickland, et al., 1991). To locate a theoretical definition, when possible we turn to the theorist who first defined the term. For example, Bandura (1997, p. 3) defined self-efficacy as "belief in one's capabilities to organize and execute the course of action required to attain a goal." And Ajzen (1991, p. 183) defined perceived behavioral control as "people's perception of the ease or difficulty of performing the behavior of interest." For a term that is not embedded in a particular theory or for which the origin is not known, we look to those who have written extensively about the concept. Among these terms are *self-esteem* and *pain*. For example, Rosenberg (1965, p. 15) is known for his work on self-esteem and defined the term as a "favorable or unfavorable opinion of oneself," an evaluation of one's worth. If we want to provide a theoretical definition of the concept of pain, we might use the definition provided by Gaston-Johnson, Fridh, and Turner-Norvell (1988), who noted that pain is a multidimensional subjective experience of discomfort composed of both sensory and affective components.

Although theoretical definitions are useful in the conceptual phrase of a study, they fail to tell us exactly how a concept will be measured in a particular study. Thus, the process of transformation includes defining the concept in the way in which it will be measured for a specific study. We refer to this type of definition as an operational (or empirical) definition, and it is the definition of the concept in terms of the manner in which it will be measured (Nunnally & Bernstein, 1994). That is, it is stated in terms of the empirical indicators that we will use to measure the concept.

Operational definitions for the concepts of self-efficacy, self-esteem, and pain might be as follows:

Self-efficacy to quit smoking will be measured by the smoking cessation self-efficacy scale.

Self-esteem will be measured by the Rosenberg Self-Esteem Scale.

Pain intensity will be measured by using a visual analog scale representing a continuum of intensity from *no pain* to *pain as bad as it can be.*

The term *operationalization* is the transformation statement found in Gibbs's model. Like the transformational statement, operationalization is the process of transforming a concept from an abstract indicator into an empirical indicator. The operationalization process includes making decisions about the way a concept will be measured, selecting the empirical indicators to be used to communicate its meaning, and selecting the procedures for measuring. In this process, based on theoretical and empirical work, the researcher or evaluator seeks to understand the meaning of the concept and the best approach to measure the concept for a specific study. Usually researchers operationalize a concept for a specific study. Two researchers might employ the same theoretical definition of a concept but choose different empirical indicators of the concept. Thus, we find operational definitions generally more restrictive and situation-specific than theoretical definitions.

Conceptualization Issues in Scale Development

Survey Versus Scale

Health behavior researchers use survey instruments to gather information about health behaviors and about the variety of factors associated with health behaviors. For example, if we are interested in motorcycle helmet use, we may want to know about the types of motorcycles people ride, how often they ride, their concerns about traffic safety, and their use of helmets. Each set of items is related to helmet use, but each set covers a different concept: type of motorcycle, riding habits, safety concerns, and helmet use. In contrast, when we develop a scale, we are interested in selecting items that measure only one concept. If we wanted to develop a scale to measure people's attitudes toward the use of motorcycle helmets, our scale would include only items related to these attitudes. It would not include items on type of motorcycle or frequency of riding a motorcycle.

Exhibit 6.1 (on pages 112 and 113) presents items written for a survey and items written for a scale. Notice that we can write the survey items in different formats with a variety of response options or short answers. Notice also that although all items are related to motorcycle or helmet use, they address different topics, including riding habits and passenger helmet use. In contrast, items written for the scale are all related to attitudes about using helmets, and all response options are the same.

Single-Item Versus Multiple-Item Scales

Spector (1992) notes that single-item assessments of concepts are unsatisfactory measures of people's opinions, attitudes, or feelings because responses to single items lack precision, tend to change over time, and are limited in scope.

Take this item related to motorcycle helmets:

People who ride motorcycles should wear helmets every time they ride.

Yes_____ No_____

Persons asked to respond to this item are forced to choose between one of two broad options, thus limiting their range of possible responses to *yes* and *no*. Other, more exact choices are not possible; thus, precision of responses is limited. The item also measures how people are feeling in general about wearing motorcycle helmets at the time when they answer the item. People who are undecided might answer favorably one day and unfavorably another day.

Multiple-item scales overcome these difficulties by expanding the number of items assessing various aspects of the concept and providing more response options. Adding items about wearing helmets under different circumstances allows people to rate helmet use on different dimensions, thus expanding the scope of the measure. By providing more options with which to rate each item, the researcher enhances precision. Rating feelings on helmet use items on a four-point agree/disagree scale allows people to rate the intensity of their feelings and provides response options for people who favor helmet use only under certain circumstances. The instrument improves the reliability or stability of responses over that of single-item measures, because a response to any one item in a scale does not overly influence the total score. For example, the total score for a person who mistakenly answers *disagree* on an item one time and later corrects that error differs by only a few points, provided that all the other responses on the scale remain the same. Scale responses also permit the categorization of people into groups based on the intensity of their feelings about helmet use, unlike single items that require a *yes* or *no* response. For example:

People who ride motorcycles should wear a helmet every time they ride.

Strongly disagree   Disagree   Agree   Strongly agree

EXHIBIT 6.1. SAMPLE SURVEY AND SCALE ITEMS, DEMONSTRATING DIFFERENCES.

Survey Items

Instructions: Please answer the following questions about motorcycle and helmet use.

What type of motorcycle do you ride? _____

How often do you ride?

_____ Daily
_____ 2–6 days/week
_____ 1–4 days/month
_____ Less than 1 day/month

How often do you wear a helmet when you ride?

_____ Every time
_____ Most of the time
_____ Sometimes
_____ Hardly ever
_____ Never

How often do you ask your passenger to wear a helmet?

_____ Every time
_____ Most of the time
_____ Sometimes
_____ Hardly ever
_____ Never

Where do you ride your motorcycle? (Check all that apply)

_____ Streets near home
_____ Side streets
_____ Dirt trails
_____ Expressway

When I ride my motorcycle, I usually ride at the speed limit or less.

_____ Yes
_____ No

Scale Items

Instructions: Please circle the word that best describes the way you feel about each of the following statements on motorcycle helmet use.

All people who ride motorcycles should wear helmets.

| Strongly disagree | Disagree | Agree | Strongly agree |

Motorcycle helmets are too hot to wear.

| Strongly disagree | Disagree | Agree | Strongly agree |

Most of my friends would make fun of me if I wore a motorcycle helmet.

| Strongly disagree | Disagree | Agree | Strongly agree |

Most people look stupid wearing motorcycle helmets.

| Strongly disagree | Disagree | Agree | Strongly agree |

Motorcycle helmets save lives.

| Strongly disagree | Disagree | Agree | Strongly agree |

Motorcycle helmets should be worn only when traveling on the expressway.

| Strongly disagree | Disagree | Agree | Strongly agree |

Concept Selection

The need for a new scale generally arises from one of two situations: no scale exists that measures the concept, or no scale exists that measures the concept in the population of interest to the researcher. Because health behavior research is a fairly new area of study and because so many concepts are available to study, the lack of a measure for a health behavior concept tends to be fairly common. In addition, our theories in health behavior often require that we develop new measures based on the behavior that we wish to study. For example, social cognitive theory requires that measures of self-efficacy be behavior-specific. If we wanted to measure individuals' degree of self-efficacy related to the use of motorcycle safety, we would first search for an instrument that measured motorcycle safety self-efficacy. If none existed, we would need to develop an appropriate self-efficacy scale before conducting the study. Other examples of theory-based constructs that require behavior-specific instruments include outcome expectations (social cognitive theory); stages of change (transtheoretical model); and perceived susceptibility, barriers, and benefits (health belief model).

A second possible reason for developing a new measure is that the existing measure of the concept is inappropriate for the intended population. For example, several measures of social support for adults exist. However, if a researcher wanted to measure social support among children and no scale existed, he or she would have to modify one developed for adults or create a new one.

Researchers need to be aware that some theoretical concepts are not amenable to measurement. A common example of a nonmeasurable concept comes from Freud's psychoanalytic theory. Because of their psychodynamic nature, the ego, id, and super-ego are not amenable to self-report measures. Likewise, though death might be a variable in some situations (for example, resuscitated, brain-dead), the afterlife is not amenable to measurement.

A researcher who accepts the challenge of developing a new measure must first select the concept and then conduct a concept analysis. The concept analysis allows the researcher to develop a solid understanding of the concept and the ways in which people use and interpret the concept. Only after the completion of the concept analysis, the clarification of the theoretical definition, and the statement of the variable should the researcher begin to write items. Because of the importance of concept analysis to the scale development process, we will devote the remainder of this chapter to a discussion of concept analysis. In Chapter Seven, we will discuss item writing.

Concept Analysis

Concept analysis is the process of developing a thorough understanding of the concept to be measured (Wilson, 1970). Scale developers should examine a variety of sources, both written and oral, for information about the concept, including its definitions, uses, and measurement. The ultimate goal of concept analysis is to clarify the meaning of the concept and its use in theory, research, and everyday life. A solid understanding of the concept and its measurement will facilitate the writing of items that reflect its essence. Using Wilson's framework, concept analysis consists of the six steps depicted in Figure 6.5.

Identify Definitions and Uses of the Concept

The concept analysis process begins with an exploration of what we know about the concept, including what theorists have written about it and how researchers have used it in their work. We gather information through reviews of the literature and media, interviews with people familiar with the concept, and personal experience. As we conduct the analysis, we record definitions, uses, measurements, contexts, and case examples.

The analysis usually begins with a literature review that identifies both theory and research that incorporate the concept. If the concept is embedded within a theory, the researcher conducts a careful examination of the theorist's writings, the definition, the use of the concept, and the context in which it is used. If more than one theory includes the concept, the researcher compares the theories, examining the meanings of the concept and its use by the theorists. The investigator also searches for studies in which the concept has been investigated. Here, it is important to learn how researchers have defined and measured the concept and how they have interpreted the results of the study. For example, more than one theory and definition exist to explain the concept of social support. Weiss (1974), for example, identified six provisions in his theory of social relationships. According to that theory, these six provisions—guidance, reliable alliance, reassurance of worth, attachment, social integration, and opportunity for nurturance—reflect what people receive from relationships with others. The six provisions were used to guide the development of the Personal Resource Questionnaire, a measure of social support (Weinert, 2003). Tilden, Nelson, and May (1990), on the other hand, have developed the Interpersonal Relationship Inventory (IPR Inventory), basing their definition of social support on social exchange and equity theories. The premise of these theories is that interactions among people are influenced by power relationships and efforts to achieve balance in relationships (Emerson, 1976).

FIGURE 6.5. STEPS IN CONDUCTING A CONCEPT ANALYSIS.

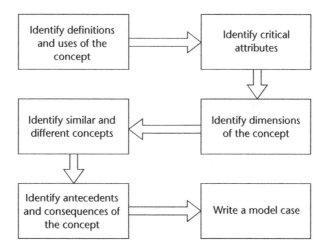

The review can also include other literature and media in which the concept appears. For example, we can use a dictionary to determine the common usage of terms, and media such as poetry, stories, art, and song to examine the portrayal of a concept.

Another approach to gathering information about a concept and its use is conducting interviews with individuals who are familiar with the concept. Investigators may conduct these interviews with individuals (that is, in unstructured or semistructured interviews) or with groups (that is, in focus groups). The purpose of the interview is to obtain information about how respondents define or understand the concept, how people use the concept, what terms they use in reference to the concept, and the context of the concept's use. Moreover, interviews help identify a greater number of contexts or situations in which the concept is used and verify or refute the use of the concept as presented in the literature and media. In addition, the researcher can call on personal experience with the concept to augment the literature review and the interviews. Researchers might be in a position to observe the concept in research, teaching, or clinical venues, and their experience can be brought to bear on the concept analysis.

Matt, as we mentioned at the beginning of this chapter, is interested in developing a scale to measure the degree to which one expects positive outcomes associated with eating a healthy diet (OE for healthy eating). We can use his example to demonstrate the concept analysis process. In reviewing the literature, Matt finds that Bandura (1997, p. 21) coined the term *outcome expectations* to refer to a person's judgment about the likely consequences of performing a specific behavior. Bandura also observed that researchers generally measure OE by first creating a set of outcomes associated with a particular behavior and then asking individuals to rate the degree to which they agree (or disagree) that a given outcome would occur if they performed the behavior. Behaviors for which OE scales have been developed include mathematical ability, career planning, chronic disease management, and sports performance. In a review of general media, including magazines, Web sites, and newspaper articles, Matt discovered that people tend to talk about outcomes associated with behaviors in everyday conversation, though they are unlikely to use the term *outcome expectations*.

Identify Critical Attributes of the Concept

To further refine the understanding of the concept, the next step in the concept analysis process is to identify the critical attributes of the concept. We scrutinize information gained from literature and media reviews, interviews with people familiar with the concept, and personal experience to isolate critical attributes. The review of the uses and definitions of the concept is likely to generate a list of characteristics that define the concept and help differentiate it from others. For example, critical attributes for the concept of OE might be anticipatory, probabilistic, and behavior-specific.

Identify Dimensions of the Concept

In the exploration of the meaning of the concept and its use in the scientific literature, the researcher also identifies any dimension of the concept and labels it important. If the concept is embedded within a theory, the theorist often identifies dimensions of the concept. Some concepts are unidimensional (having only one dimension), whereas others are multidimensional (including more than one aspect). Although all aspects, or dimensions, refer to the overarching concept, each aspect is slightly different. For example, Fitts (1965), in his discussion of self-concept, noted five dimensions: physical, moral, personal, family, and social. An instrument developed to measure self-concept using his definition would likely include items to measure these five different aspects.

Matt has observed that Bandura (1997) identified three dimensions of OE: (1) self-evaluative, (2) social, and (3) physical OE. If we talk about OE related to running a marathon, self-evaluative OE might include feeling proud of one's accomplishment; social OE might include accolades from friends and family; and physical OE might include the prospect of dehydration, sore muscles, and a leaner body. In regard to OE for healthy eating, people might expect that they would feel that they were doing the right thing for their health, that their doctors would approve of their diet, and that their cholesterol levels would remain low.

Identify Similar and Different Concepts

One of the goals of the concept analysis process is to identify concepts that are similar in meaning to the chosen concept and those that are different from it. An evaluation of the attributes that make the concepts similar but slightly different advances the researcher's understanding of the concept and helps him or her clarify the meaning of the concept before writing items to measure it. Similar concepts are those that possess some but not all of the attributes of the chosen concept; different concepts are those that possess none of its attributes. Comparing and contrasting the meanings of similar, related, and different concepts help the researcher to further understand how the chosen concepts fit within a group of concepts.

A concept similar to that of OE is subjective norms, a concept within the theory of planned behavior. Fishbein and Ajzen (1975) define subjective norms as people's perceptions of the social pressure related to performing or not performing a behavior. As we have learned, OE has a social component, defined as the outcomes one would expect for others if the behavior were performed. An item such as "If I ate a healthy diet, my doctor would approve" could function as an OE item because it reflects the critical attributes of OE. It is behavior-specific, anticipatory, and probabilistic. The item "My doctor thinks I should eat a healthy diet" can be classified as a subjective-norm item, but not as an OE item. This latter statement is a perception of the opinion of another, but not a perceived outcome of a behavior. Benefits and barriers—concepts within the health belief model—are also similar to the concept of OE. Both are behavior-specific. However, though some benefits and barriers might be outcomes of performing a behavior, there is no requirement that all benefits and barriers be related to outcomes, a condition of OE.

Concepts that possess none of the critical attributes associated with OE might include depression, fame, and stigma.

Identify Antecedents and Consequences of the Concept

We can identify the antecedents and consequences of the selected concept by reviewing the literature and through discussions with others. Antecedents are events, actions, processes, cognitions, or feelings that occur before the expression of the concept. In the case of OE, Bandura (1997) notes that there are four primary sources of efficacy information, which in turn influence one's expectations of outcomes associated with a behavior. The four sources of efficacy information are enactment of the behavior, vicarious learning, verbal persuasion, and physical or affective states related to the performance. For example, surrounding oneself with others who eat well can increase one's chances of developing positive expectations about healthy eating. Consequences are those events, actions, processes, cognitions, or feelings that follow the expression of the concept. A person who expects positive outcomes to be associated with maintaining a healthy diet is likely to be successful in altering his or her eating habits to achieve this goal despite previous failed attempts. These positive feelings about a healthy diet are likely to motivate the person to eat well and perhaps to spark an interest in looking for low-fat recipes. In contrast, a person who expects that it will be difficult to maintain a diet low in fat and high in fruits and vegetables might struggle to change his or her eating habits, give up quickly, and fail to achieve the goal.

Write a Model Case

The final step in the concept analysis process is to write an exemplar that demonstrates the critical attributes of the concept. Below is a model case that Matt wrote for the concept of OE for healthy eating.

Mary is a seventy-eight-year-old woman who is in reasonably good health. She has hypertension, controlled by daily medications, and arthritis in her knees and hips. She has no other health problems, but is about 20 pounds overweight. She walks every day and goes to the gym three or four times per week. Here she uses the treadmill, lifts weights, and uses the weight machines for upper-body strength. She lives alone and does not always eat as well as she should. Some of her dinners consist of snacking on high-fat foods. She believes that if she changed her diet by lowering her fat intake and increasing the number of fruits and vegetables that she eats every day, she would lose some weight and her knees would not hurt as much when she walks. She also thinks that she could lower her blood pressure and not have to take an extra water pill every three days. Her children have encouraged her to eat better, and she knows that they would approve of her changing her diet. She also believes that a diet change is what she needs to do for her health. In making changes in her diet, Mary is aware that her expectations of these positive outcomes will keep her motivated to continue despite the fact that it will take some extra effort to prepare wholesome meals.

State the Variables

Following the concept analysis, it is important to state a concept in the form of a variable before beginning the item-writing process. Although we all know that a variable is a concept or construct that takes on different values for different people under the same conditions (that is, it varies), a more precise definition that is useful in making relational statements is, "A variable is a set of values, only to one of which can an object ever be assigned at any one time" (Mulaik, 2004, page 428). For example, the values of a marital status variable might be *never married, married, divorced, separated,* and *widowed.* A person can be assigned to only one of these values at any one time.

Mulaik (2004) notes that constructs such as self-efficacy, locus of control, self-concept, patient satisfaction, and quality of life as stated are not variables because it is not evident from these terms what varies. To create variables from these and similar constructs, a researcher must understand what quantity is being measured. A precisely defined variable is stated in terms of quantities such as "degrees to which," "frequency with which," and "amount to which" (Mulaik, 2004). Moreover, variables are unidimensional in that they vary on only one attribute.

For example, as stated, the concept *patient satisfaction* does not give us a clue as to what precisely is being measured. Is the researcher interested in how much the patient is satisfied with his or her care? How often patients are satisfied with care? The degree to which the patient is satisfied with access to care, communication with the doctor, nursing care, or cost of care? The concept analysis process helps the researcher understand the meaning of the concept, and the statement of the concept in terms of a variable clarifies precisely what is being measured.

Summary

As can be seen from the discussion in this chapter, a carefully conducted concept analysis will provide health educators and behavioral scientists with a thorough understanding of concepts that they seek to measure. The task of writing items for scales becomes much easier when the scale developer, before attempting to write items, thoroughly understands the concept and how it is the same as and different from other concepts. Knowing the subtle differences that distinguish concepts facilitates more efficient item writing and will save the researcher considerable work in the assessment of reliability and validity, which we will discuss in Chapters Nine, Ten, and Eleven. In this chapter, we have presented only a summary of the concept analysis process. Readers who are developing scales may desire more information. They are encouraged to read Chinn and Kramer (1995), Walker and Avant (1988), and Wilson (1970).

CHAPTER SEVEN

ITEM WRITING AND SCALING

LEARNING OBJECTIVES

At the end of this chapter, the student should be able to

1. Identify the steps in the item development process.
2. Create a matrix for writing scale items.
3. List three ways to obtain information for writing items.
4. Identify three issues associated with item writing for summated rating scales.

In Chapter Six, we discussed procedures for analyzing concepts. We learned that a thorough concept analysis should conclude with a statement of the theoretical definition and a description of the attributes associated with the concept. Moreover, the concept should be stated in the form of a variable to clearly identify the quantity that is being measured. This information is then used to guide the item-writing process, which we discuss in this chapter. In this chapter, we present the steps (or plan) used to develop a set of items that together measure a variable as defined by the researcher. We also address some specific scale development issues related to summated rating scales (that is, Likert scales). We must be mindful, as Nunnally and Bernstein (1994, p. 297) say, that a "good plan represents an intention to construct a good test, but unless items are skillfully written, the plan never materializes." Although in this chapter we will not discuss the characteristics of items themselves, this information can be found in Chapters Four and Five. Many of the characteristics of writing survey, multiple-choice, and true/false items are also part of writing items for scales.

Item Development Process

The item-writing process consists of the following six steps, which are shown in Figure 7.1:

1. State the theoretical definition.
2. Identify the dimensions of the concept.
3. Create a content-domain by concept-dimension matrix.
4. Decide how many items to include for each cell in the matrix.
5. Write items for each content-domain by concept-dimension cell in the matrix.
6. Write the rules for the scoring and administration of the scale.

Following we describe each of these steps, using as an example items written for a scale measuring the concept *outcome expectations for healthy eating.*

FIGURE 7.1. STEPS IN THE ITEM-WRITING PROCESS.

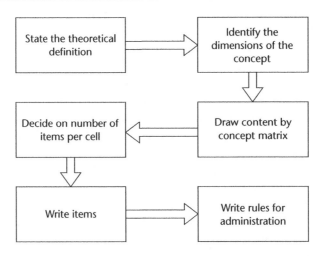

State the Theoretical Definition

To begin the item-writing process, the researcher refers to the theoretical definition and the attributes of the concept derived from the concept analysis. For example, using the definition of outcome expectations presented by Bandura (1997), we define the concept *outcome expectations for healthy eating* as those outcomes one expects if one eats a diet low in saturated fat and high in fruits and vegetables. This definition suggests that the researcher is interested in outcomes associated with eating a healthy diet and has identified three content domains:—eating a low-fat diet, eating fruits, and eating vegetables. The researcher could combine these three behaviors and call the combination a healthy diet, or could conceptualize each behavior separately. In the example that appears later, the three behaviors are treated as three content domains of a healthy diet.

Identify Dimensions of the Concept

If, during the concept analysis, the researcher determines that the concept is composed of more than one dimension (is multidimensional, as opposed to unidimensional), the dimensions can be treated separately. For our example of OE, we find that Bandura (1997) conceptualized three dimensions of OE: (1) self-evaluative OE, (2) social OE, and (3) physical OE. Self-evaluative OE consists of those outcomes one expects to personally experience if one performs the behavior. Social OE consists of those outcomes that one expects others to experience if one performs the behavior. Physical OE, of course, consists of those outcomes that are physical in nature. If we apply these dimensions to OE for healthy eating, we might conclude that eating a healthy diet would result in the following: (1) feeling good about oneself (self-evaluative OE), (2) gaining the approval of others (social OE), and (3) maintaining a desired weight (physical OE).

Create a Content-Domain by Concept-Dimension Matrix

For ease of item development, the researcher creates a matrix (also called a blueprint) that visually displays the content to be addressed by the items and the dimensions of the concept that will be measured. This matrix is similar to the table of test specifications for knowledge tests (Table 5.1) that we discussed in Chapter Five. The simplest matrix is composed of one content domain for a unidimensional concept (a concept with only one dimension). Table 7.1 shows the matrix for a scale to measure barriers to the use of sun protection products. Here, the researcher is interested in writing only items related to an individual's opinion of the physical and psychosocial costs of using sunscreen products. All the items developed for this scale must correspond to the definition of barriers and be specific to sun protection products.

TABLE 7.1. EXAMPLE OF A 1 × 1 MATRIX.

Content	Sunscreen Product Use
Barriers	

If the researcher wanted to develop items for the eight dimensions of social capital using Bullen and Onyx's (2005) framework, the matrix would consist of one row and eight columns, as shown in Table 7.2. A matrix for the concept of OE related to healthy eating using the three content dimensions of low fat, fruits, and vegetables would look like that in Table 7.3. In this matrix, we see the content domains of the concept of a healthy diet along the left side (low fat, fruits, and vegetables), and the dimensions of the concept OE across the top (self-evaluative, social, and physical). When preparing the matrix, it is important to identify the variable for each cell. Being explicit about the quantity to measure will assist with writing items. For example, for the social capital dimension of community participation, we would write the variable as "the extent to which one joins local community organizations."

Decide How Many Items to Include for Each Matrix Cell

The matrix helps the researcher visualize the content domains and the concept dimensions. It also helps the researcher identify the number and type of items required to adequately measure the concept. Thus, the next step in the item-writing process is to use the matrix as a guide to determine how many items to write for each cell in the matrix. In our example of OE for healthy eating, the researcher might decide to write five items for each cell, in which case the final scale would contain forty-five items. As we discussed earlier in Chapter Six, Matt is creating such a scale for men and women over age sixty-five. Generally, long scales are difficult for elderly people to complete. Thus, Matt must make some decisions about how many items to include for each of the cells. If Matt believes that a forty-five-item scale is too long, he can write fewer items for each cell. Alternatively, he might believe that the measurement of OE related to fruits and vegetables is more important than that of OE related to low fat. In that case, he will write more items to assess fruits and vegetables and fewer to assess low fat. Likewise, if Matt believes that personal OE is more important to measure than physical OE, he can write more items to assess the personal dimension of OE than items to address the physical dimension.

Generally, researchers write more items than needed for a scale. In the process of evaluating the scale for reliability and validity, most likely some items will not fare well and will be deleted. To guard against having fewer items than desired for the final scale, it is important to include a sufficient number in the original pool.

TABLE 7.2. EXAMPLE OF AN 8 × 1 MATRIX.

Content	Community Participation	Trust	Tolerance	Neighborhood Connections	Family and Friend Connections	Work Connections	Value of Life	Proactivity in Social Context
Social Capital								

TABLE 7.3. MATRIX FOR OUTCOME EXPECTATIONS FOR HEALTHY EATING.

Dimensions for Outcome Expectations for Healthy Eating

Content Domain	Self-Evaluative	Social	Physical
Low fat			
Fruits			
Vegetables			

Write Items for Each Content-Domain by Concept-Dimension Cell

The matrix guides the researcher in determining the content areas and the number of items to write, but for the actual phrasing of items, the researcher turns to other sources. These include (1) experts (literature review or personal contacts), (2) qualitative interviews with representatives of the population, and (3) other measuring instruments.

Literature Review. During the process of concept analysis, the researcher likely collected examples of phrases from the literature that embodied the concept. These phrases now become useful in developing items. For example, in reading about the reasons why people choose to eat well, the researcher might discover that people want to maintain an acceptable weight, to have more energy, to lose weight so that their clothes fit better, to receive the approval of family and friends, and to live longer. We can transform each of these facts into an item to measure OE:

> If I ate a low-fat diet, I would maintain my weight.
>
> If I ate a low-fat diet, I would have more energy.
>
> If I ate a low-fat diet, I would lose weight.
>
> If I ate a low-fat diet, my clothes would fit better.
>
> If I ate a low-fat diet, my family would be pleased.
>
> If I ate a low-fat diet, I would live longer.

Note that the first and third items are very similar. Matt might include only one of these items in the scale at this point in the development process, or he might keep both items and determine which is the better item after reliability and validity assessments have been completed.

Qualitative Interviews. Information collected from members of the population in which the concept appears, through either focus groups or qualitative interviews, provides another rich source of phrases for the generation of items. For example, suppose Matt conducted a focus group to find out what elderly men and women eat, what barriers they face in eating a healthy diet, and what they believe are its benefits.

In one focus group, Matt says to the group: "So far, we have discussed what we think a healthy diet is. You mentioned that eating less fat would be considered part of a healthy diet. This might include eating only one or two servings of red meat per week and not snacking on potato chips and cookies. Now I would like to ask you what you think are some of the benefits of eating a low-fat diet."

Respondent 1: "I have high blood pressure. Every time I go to my doctor, she tells me to eat less fat. She thinks that if I did, my blood pressure would go down, and I would not have to take so many pills."

Respondent 2: "They say that eating fat will make cholesterol build up in the arteries near your heart and that when the cholesterol builds up there, it can block the arteries and cause a heart attack. So if you eat less meat and more vegetables, you have less chance of having a heart attack. I am trying to eat more vegetables because my mother and her sister both had heart attacks in their fifties."

Respondent 3: "I really, really like chocolate, and it is hard for me not to eat it. But if I stopped eating it and ate fruit instead, I would probably be able to lose some weight. If I could lose 20 pounds, I would feel a lot better."

In this exchange, each of these respondents revealed an expectation about an outcome he or she might realize if he or she ate a healthy diet. In constructing items, we can draw on their comments. For example:

If I ate a low-fat diet, my blood pressure would go down.

If I ate vegetables, I would be less likely to have a heart attack.

If I ate fruits, I would lose weight.

Other Instruments. In addition to talking with members of the population, researchers can review other instruments to locate useful items during the development of the new scale. They can obtain scales from other researchers, from written sources such as books and journal articles, from companies that sell the instruments, and from Internet sources. Before using an item, researchers should first determine its copyright status and obtain permission from the developer of the instrument. Once it is obtained, they must review items to determine their fit with the purpose of the new scale and with the theoretical definition. Researchers may include items as written or they may modify them to fit the scale.

Recall that in Matt's first attempt to develop an OE scale, he did not have the benefit of information obtained from a concept analysis. Thus, he and the staff members relied on their own interpretations of the concept to generate items for the scale. Sometimes this approach works, particularly if the researcher is the same person who identified the concept. (For example, Bandura [1997] identified the construct of self-efficacy and then taught people how to measure it.) Most of the time, however, a scale developed without sufficient understanding of the concept will demonstrate problems during reliability and validity testing, which we will discuss in Chapters Ten and Eleven.

One person or several people can write items for a scale. If more than one person is involved in item writing, all the item writers should understand the variable and agree on its meaning. Ideally, all the item writers have involved themselves in the concept analysis and the generation of the theoretical definition and attributes for the concept and the statement of the variable. Following the creation of the definition, the group writes several sample items. They review the sample items for consistency with the conceptual definition. After the members of the group agree on the final forms of these sample items, they assign each member to write items according to the matrix. After the items are complete, the group convenes to discuss and modify them until members agree that the items adequately measure the variable, and they express satisfaction with the phrasing of the items. During the testing of the scale, researchers identify and delete weak items, leaving only those that have functioned well during the testing process.

Write Rules for Scale Scoring and Administration

The final task in scale development is to write rules for scoring items and administering the scale to respondents. Rules for scoring scale items correspond to the type of scale used. In Chapter Two, we presented a description of five types of scales:—VAS, Thurstone, Guttman, semantic differential, and Likert. Because the Likert scale (also called a summated rating scale) is the most common type of scale used in health behavior research, we will describe the scoring rules for the Likert scale in the section that follows. Though scoring rules depend on the type of scale, rules for administration depend on the preferences of the scale developer and, to some extent, correspond to the medium used to present the scale and the data collection procedures. For example, a seven-point scale might be used for scale items that participants complete using paper and pencil. In contrast, the developer might consider using three to five response options for scale items presented to participants over the telephone. Scale developers may have preferences about the order of the items, the type of response options, the use of adjectives, adverbs, or numbers on the response scale, and the format for presentation. These preferences are included in the description of the scale.

Summated Rating Scales

Types of Response Options

To construct a Likert scale, Rensis Likert (1932), who first described this type of summated rating scale, suggested developing a pool of statements reflecting different views about an attribute. He said that each statement should express a desired behavior rather than a statement of fact and suggested using items with the word *should* as well as items that are "clear, concise, and straightforward" (Likert, 1932, p. 45). Likert's original scale consisted of statements and the following five response options for each statement: *strongly approve, approve, undecided, disapprove,* and *strongly disapprove.*

Today, response options are designed to represent graduated increments of agreement, frequency, or evaluation (Spector, 1992). Using a scale that assesses agreement, respondents indicate how much they agree with a particular statement; for frequency, respondents indicate how often they perform a particular behavior; and for the evaluative scale, respondents rate items according to how positively or negatively they feel about what is described. The choices for response options include *agree/disagree; never/always; never/very often; never true/always true;* and *not at all sure/very sure.* The researcher should select the type of scale (agreement, frequency, evaluative) that corresponds to the statement of the variable. Ideally, the wording of the response options is selected before writing the items. However, because of the dynamic nature of the item-writing process, a researcher might want to make the final decision on the response options after a draft of some or most of the items has been written. If researchers delay the decision, they must review the items to make sure respondents can answer them on the selected response scale (Exhibit 7.1).

EXHIBIT 7.1. EXAMPLES OF RESPONSE OPTIONS.

Agreement				
Strongly disagree	Disagree	Neither agree nor disagree	Agree	Strongly agree
Not at all true	Somewhat untrue	Somewhat true	Very true	

Evaluation					
Not at all important	Unimportant	Somewhat unimportant	Somewhat important	Important	Very important
Most unpleasant	Unpleasant	Neutral	Pleasant	Most pleasant	
Not at all sure	Somewhat sure	Very sure			

Frequency				
Never	Almost never	Sometimes	Most of the time	Always
Not at all	Occasionally	Frequently	Regularly	

If words are being used as response options, the researcher needs to decide on the terminology for rating each item. As noted above, the researcher has several choices, including *agree/disagree, never/always, never true/always true,* and *not at all sure/very sure.* Regardless of the response options, it is important to read each item to make certain the items are consistent with the response choices. In the first example below, the question cannot reasonably be answered with the response options given. The item makes more sense using the second set of response options.

How often do you wear a helmet when you ride a motorcycle?

Strongly agree   Agree   Neither   Disagree   Strongly disagree

How often do you wear a helmet when you ride a motorcycle?

Every time   Most of the time   Sometimes   Hardly ever   Never

Number of Response Options

Likert (1932) originally proposed five response choices for attitudinal items, ranging from *strongly disapprove* to *strongly approve.* However, today the number of options can vary from three to ten. Although theoretically we can provide more than ten choices, most people find it difficult to discriminate among more than seven options (Streiner & Norman, 1995). Occasionally a researcher uses a scale labeled from 0 to 100. In this case, the scale is usually calibrated in units of 10, so that in reality, no more than eleven choices are available. For example:

Rate your level of confidence with the following statement:

How sure are you that you can always exercise three times per week for thirty minutes each time?

0   10   20   30   40   50   60   70   80   90   100

Not at all sure   Very sure

We could also show the scale in this way:

0   1   2   3   4   5   6   7   8   9   10

Not at all sure   Very sure

The number of response options depends on several considerations, including the age of the respondent, the experience of the respondent with this type of rating scale, the ability of the respondent to discriminate between options, the preference of the researcher, and the content of the scale. Respondents who are very young, are very old, or have low literacy have difficulty discriminating among more than two or three options. Thus, limiting response options to two choices, such as *yes/no* or *agree/disagree*, makes it easier for members of these populations to answer. The same is true for individuals who have no experience in answering items using Likert-type scales. The novelty of the scale is likely to interfere with their responding accurately to the items.

As noted above, the ability to discriminate between options is an important consideration. Items that include only *yes* and *no* as possible responses fail to allow room for discrimination. Thus, individuals who might agree that motorcycle helmets should be worn under certain conditions (such as while riding on the highway) might have difficulty responding to the following item:

People who ride motorcycles should wear helmets.

Expanding the number of response options to five, with anchors of *strongly agree* and *strongly disagree*, allows respondents more choices. Expanding the response options further, to seven, may offset the tendency of some participants to avoid selecting the extreme (or end) options (Streiner & Norman, 1995). In addition, research has shown that scales using few response options have lower internal-consistency reliability than those with more. The difference is due to the lack of precision and the loss of information that occur when respondents are given an insufficient number of response choices (Spector, 1992). Based on research studies and experience, the most common recommendation is that scales include between five and seven response choices.

Odd or Even Number of Categories

Another issue raised repeatedly among researchers is whether to use an odd or even number of response options. For agreement and evaluative rating scales, the middle category suggests a neutral point or a *don't know* response. For example:

People who ride motorcycles should wear helmets.
Strongly agree   Agree   Neither agree nor disagree   Disagree   Strongly disagree

A person who does not have strong opinions might choose the middle category, as would a person who is unfamiliar with the value of motorcycle helmets. Researchers differ in their opinions about how to analyze and interpret this middle category. Some suggest deleting all respondents who choose the middle category or including them in the analyses as a separate group. Others consider the middle category to be the midpoint of a continuum between *agree* and *disagree*.

The use of an even number of categories, as shown below, forces respondents to choose an *agree* or *disagree* option and avoids the need to make decisions about how data will be treated for analysis and interpretation.

People who ride motorcycles should wear helmets.

Strongly agree   Agree   Disagree   Strongly disagree

Meanings of Response Option Adjectives or Adverbs

Some research examines the ways in which people interpret adjectives or adverbs that label options on the response scale (Ostrom & Gannon, 1996; Schaeffer, 1991). A frequency scale, for example, might include the following adverbs: *never, rarely, sometimes, often, most of the time,* and *always.* Research has shown that people interpret these adverbs differently. For some people, the terms *sometimes* and *often* are closer in their interpretations than the terms *often* and *most of the time.* The researcher might make the assumption that these adverbs represent equal intervals, as shown here:

Never   Rarely   Sometimes   Often   Most of the time

Other respondents might interpret the adverbs as representing unequal intervals, in this way:

Never   Rarely   Sometimes   Often   Most of the time

In a related issue, respondents may disagree on the interpretation of the words themselves due to the vagueness of the terms. So, when responding to an item, people will respond with their own interpretations—what the item means to them—at the time. Obviously, the researchers will not be aware of these interpretations when they analyze the data and will make assumptions about how people interpreted the items. In Chapter Eleven, we will discuss cognitive assessment as a method to evaluate items to determine how people are interpreting them. Information from this type of assessment can help the researcher improve the statement of items before completing the final scale.

Use of Adjectives, Adverbs, or Numbers, or Combinations Thereof

In developing a scale, a researcher must decide whether to use words or numbers or both as response options. We know that adjective and adverb descriptors are generally vague and that respondents interpret the words differently. Using numbers may help people decide on the degree to which they endorse a particular item. In U.S. society, we commonly use the 1-to-10 verbal scale. ("On a 1-to-10 scale, how would you rate . . . .?") In this instance, adding numbers or using numbers with adjectives or adverbs might help people with the task of determining their levels of agreement or their opinions. Schwarz and colleagues (1991), however, found that the values of the numbers associated with adjectives can make a difference in the ways people respond. In their study, participants were asked to complete the same eleven-point scale with the extremes labeled *not at all successful* and *extremely successful*. Half the participants received scales whose response options were labeled with numbers from −5 to +5; for the other half, the response options were labeled from 0 to 10. Only 13 percent of participants responding to items using the −5 to +5 scale selected responses at the lower end of the scale (−5 to 0), whereas 34 percent of participants in the other group selected responses at the lower end when the scale ranged between 0 and 5. This study shows that people do use numbers in addition to interpretations of adjectives to make decisions about their responses (Streiner & Norman, 1994).

Positively and Negatively Worded Items

To encourage attention to the task and reduce the tendency for response sets such as yea-saying, Likert (1932) suggested that about half the items be presented in a positive way and the other half in a negative way. The typical Likert scale, such as the Rosenberg Self-Esteem Scale, follows this convention (see Table 2.1 in Chapter Two). And though it is a good rule to follow, the negative statements themselves can be a source of respondent measurement error if they include words such as *not* or *never* or prefixes such as *un-*. In Chapter Four, we indicated that one of the rules of item writing was to use negative words sparingly and, when one is used, to highlight it in the item statement. The reason is that respondents who are using a satisficing approach to complete a scale can misread the negative words and answer incorrectly. If a negatively worded item is used, the item should be phrased in such a way that words such as *not* are avoided. For example, the item, "I did not take my medications yesterday," could be rewritten as, "I missed my medications yesterday."

Another issue with negatively worded items is that some concepts and response scales do not lend themselves very well to negative statements. Bandura (1997) recommends that self-efficacy items be positive statements because of the awkward wording needed to meet the requirement of negatively worded items. Consider the following item: The participant is asked to rate his or her level of confidence on a scale from 0, *not confident at all*, to 10, *very confident that I can do:* "I can always walk outside, even when it is raining." The same statement, worded negatively, might be, "I do not walk outside when it is raining." Despite the negative wording, the item cannot be answered using the confidence rating scale because the interpretation of the item would change.

Scoring

To create a total score for a summated rating scale, responses to individual items are summed. Some researchers use the total score in analyses; others elect to compute a mean score. The latter method converts the total score into the units used to rate the individual items (that is, 1 to 4 or 1 to 5) and is sometimes helpful when the researcher compares scores from several scales. When summing responses to individual items, the researcher must reverse-score the negatively worded items so that the total score reflects a greater amount or degree of the concept. (See Chapters Two and Eight.) To demonstrate the scoring for a Likert scale, the OE scale for healthy eating is presented in Table 7.4. There are twelve items, each rated on a four-point rating scale from *strongly disagree* to *strongly agree*. Total scores are found by summing responses to individual items. The possible total scores for this scale range from 12 to 48. A high score reflects more positive outcomes associated with eating a healthy diet.

TABLE 7.4. ITEMS ON THE OUTCOME EXPECTATIONS FOR HEALTHY EATING SCALE.

Below is a list of statements about things that might happen if you were to eat a healthy diet. A healthy diet is one that is low in fat and high in fruits and vegetables.

Circle the number from 1 to 4 that most closely fits with how much you agree with each statement. If you strongly disagree, circle 1. If you disagree with the statement, circle 2. If you agree, circle 3. If you strongly agree, circle 4.

Statement	Strongly Disagree	Disagree	Agree	Strongly Agree
1. If you eat a healthy diet, you will have more energy.	1	2	3	4
2. If you eat a healthy diet, you will feel better about yourself.	1	2	3	4
3. If you eat a healthy diet, you will live longer.	1	2	3	4
4. If you eat a healthy diet, your best friends will approve.	1	2	3	4
5. If you eat a healthy diet, you will feel more responsible.	1	2	3	4
6. If you eat a healthy diet, you will control your weight.	1	2	3	4
7. If you eat a healthy diet, you will feel proud of yourself.	1	2	3	4
8. If you eat a healthy diet, you will be less likely to have a stroke.	1	2	3	4
9. If you eat a healthy diet, your friends will be proud of you.	1	2	3	4
10. If you eat a healthy diet, you will feel you are doing the right thing.	1	2	3	4
11. If you eat a healthy diet, your doctor will approve.	1	2	3	4
12. If you eat a healthy diet, your close relatives will approve.	1	2	3	4

Summary

This chapter has been devoted to a discussion of the steps necessary to write items for scales. The process begins with a statement of the theoretical definition, which is used to guide writing items that are consistent with both the content domains and the dimensions denoted by the concept. A content-domain by concept-dimension matrix helps the scale developer visualize the task and ensures that an adequate number of items are written to measure both the content and any dimensions of the concept. Upon completion of the item-writing task, the scale developer stipulates the rules for scoring and for administration of the scale in research or evaluation studies.

CHAPTER EIGHT

REVIEW OF STATISTICAL CONCEPTS

LEARNING OBJECTIVES

At the end of this chapter, the student should be able to

1. Describe the characteristics of a correlation.
2. Use SPSS to run a correlation between two variables.
3. Interpret a correlation between two variables.
4. Describe a correlation matrix.
5. Discuss issues of causality, sample size, group differences, and restriction of range related to correlations.
6. Describe the characteristics of variance.
7. Calculate variance.
8. Interpret variance.
9. List the uses of ANOVA.
10. Use SPSS to conduct an ANOVA.
11. Interpret the results of an ANOVA.

After a scale is constructed, it must be assessed for reliability and validity prior to widespread use. Reliability and validity procedures are based on statistical concepts—in particular, correlation analyses. To evaluate instruments, researchers must have a good understanding of how to conduct a correlation analysis and how to interpret the results. Some tests of validity also require an understanding of analysis of variance.

Before delving into specific psychometric tests, we present in this chapter a brief review of the principles of correlation and ANOVA. We begin the chapter with a review of frequency distributions and end with a description and example of one-way ANOVA. To foster understanding, we include the computation for correlations. However, because computer software programs are most likely to be used in practice, we include the commands for conducting the statistical tests using SPSS statistical software. In presenting the material, we assume that most students have had a course in statistics and are able to use this chapter as a review of the material. We also assume that the student has some familiarity with SPSS or another statistical software program.

Basic Statistical Concepts

Before discussing correlation and ANOVA, we review frequency distributions, measures of central tendency, and measures of dispersion.

Frequency Distribution

The first step in most statistical analyses is to examine the scores of participants on each variable. The best way to examine scores is to create a frequency distribution, which presents the number and percentage of participants for each score on the variable. Consider the distribution of scores presented in Table 8.1. These are the responses of 100 individuals participating in a hypothetical study to promote exercise and healthy eating. The participants were asked to use an eleven-point response scale to rate the degree to which they believed they would benefit from an exercise program. The scale values range from 0, *no benefit at all,* to 10, *benefit a great deal.* The benefit ratings are shown in the column on the left. The second column presents the number of participants who selected each value, and the next column gives the percentage of participants who selected each value. The column on the right provides the cumulative percentage, which is computed by adding each successive percentage. We can see that five (5 percent) participants did not believe an exercise program would be beneficial and that eleven (11 percent) believed that they would benefit a great deal from their programs of exercise. Forty-eight percent rated their perceived benefit at 5 or lower on the scale.

A frequency distribution of these data can be presented graphically as shown in Figure 8.1. Here, the benefit ratings of the 100 participants are graphed. In this bar graph, the benefit ratings are presented on the *x*-axis, and the number (or frequency) of respondents who marked each score is presented on the *y*-axis.

TABLE 8.1. FREQUENCY AND PERCENTAGE OF PARTICIPANTS' BENEFIT RATINGS (*N* = 100).

Benefit Rating	Frequency	Percentage	Cumulative Percentage
0	5	5.0	5.0
1	6	6.0	11.0
2	9	9.0	20.0
3	7	7.0	27.0
4	11	11.0	38.0
5	10	10.0	48.0
6	8	8.0	56.0
7	10	10.0	66.0
8	11	11.0	77.0
9	12	12.0	89.0
10	11	11.0	100.0
Total	100	100.0	

FIGURE 8.1. GRAPHIC REPRESENTATION OF BENEFIT RATINGS FOR A SAMPLE OF 100 PARTICIPANTS.

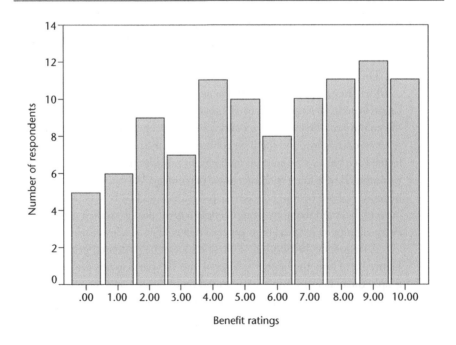

Benefit ratings

Measures of Central Tendency. Frequency distributions can be measurement of central tendency and dispersion. As you learned in your basic statistics class, there are three types of central tendency: the mean, the median, and the mode. Measures of central tendency give an estimate of the center of the distribution. The mean is the average of all the scores in the distribution and is found by adding the scores and dividing by the number of scores. The mean is considered a relatively stable statistic. However, it is affected more than the mode or the median by extreme scores. The median is the score that divides a distribution in half so that 50 percent of the scores are above the median score and 50 percent are below. The median score can easily be located in a distribution whose scores are arranged in order from high to low. For an odd number of scores, the median is the middle score, and for an even number of scores, the median is the average of the two middle scores. The median is preferable as an index of central tendency when a distribution is highly skewed or asymmetrical. The mode is the most frequently occurring score in the distribution. Some distributions will have more than one mode—two or more scores that occur at the same frequency.

Consider the distribution of scores presented in Table 8.1. The mean, calculated by summing the responses and dividing by 100, is 5.63. The median can be found by examining the cumulative percentage column. This shows that the score of 6 marks the point at which 50 percent of the scores are higher. The mode, in this case 9, is the most frequently occurring score: twelve respondents chose 9 as their benefit rating.

Measures of Dispersion. Another aspect of distributions is dispersion, or variability. The term *dispersion* refers to the spread of scores. Three types of dispersion are range, variance, and standard deviation. The range is the difference between the highest and lowest scores in the distribution. The variance is the average squared distance of scores from the mean and is calculated using the following formula.

Equation 8.1

$$s^2 = \frac{\Sigma(X - \overline{X})^2}{N - 1}$$

where

s^2 = variance,
Σ = sigma, which indicates to sum what follows
X = score on the item,
$\overline{X}$ = mean of the set of scores, and
N = number of observations.

Restated in words, to calculate the variance of a distribution, the mean is subtracted from each score and the resulting value is squared. The sum of the squared deviations from the mean is divided by one less than the total number of observations to yield the variance.

Because it is difficult to interpret squared units of a variable, taking the square root converts the variance into the standard deviation. The standard deviation is the average distance of scores from the mean and is expressed in the same units as the original measure.

Equation 8.2

$$s = \sqrt{s^2}$$

where

s = the standard deviation, and
s^2 = the variance.

For the scores presented in Table 8.1, the range is the difference between the low score of 0 and the high score of 10, which is ten points. The calculation of variance for this distribution of scores is presented in Table 8.2. In this table, the first column on the left shows the benefit rating, the second column shows the number of respondents for each rating, the third column shows the numbers inserted into the variance formula, and the final column shows the results of subtracting the mean from each score, squaring the difference, and multiplying by the number of respondents for each rating. The sum of the squared deviations is 915.32. To calculate the variance, 915.32 is divided by 99 to obtain the variance of 9.24. The standard deviation of 3.04 is obtained by taking the square root of 9.24.

$$s^2 = \frac{915.32}{99} = 9.24.$$

$$s = \sqrt{9.24} = 3.04.$$

Using this information, we can say that the distribution of benefit ratings ranges from 0 to 10, with a mean of 5.63 and a standard deviation of 3.04.

SPSS Commands

In this chapter, we introduce the SPSS commands to generate descriptive and parametric statistics that are used in reliability and validity analysis. We assume that the student is familiar with SPSS or a similar Windows-based statistical software package. If you are not familiar with statistical software, you can skip these sections or learn

TABLE 8.2. CALCULATION OF VARIANCE USING BENEFIT RATINGS OF 100 PARTICIPANTS.

Benefit Rating	N	$N(X - \overline{X})^2$	$N(X - \overline{X})^2$
0	5	$5(0 - 5.63)^2$	158.48
1	6	$6(1 - 5.63)^2$	128.62
2	9	$9(2 - 5.63)^2$	118.59
3	7	$7(3 - 5.63)^2$	48.42
4	11	$11(4 - 5.63)^2$	29.23
5	10	$10(5 - 5.63)^2$	3.97
6	8	$8(6 - 5.63)^2$	1.10
7	10	$10(7 - 5.63)^2$	18.77
8	11	$11(8 - 5.63)^2$	61.79
9	12	$12(9 - 5.63)^2$	136.28
10	11	$11(10 - 5.63)^2$	210.07
Sum		$\sum N(X - \overline{X})^2$	915.32

Sum of the squared deviations from the mean

basic information by reading the *SPSS 13.0 Base User's Manual* (SPSS, 2004) or a how-to manual such as *How to Use SPSS* (Cronk, 1999).

Throughout this book, we use the same format in presenting SPSS commands. Briefly, all commands begin from the Data Editor Screen (Figure 8.2). Across the top of the Data Editor Screen are headings indicating procedures for managing and analyzing data. We will usually begin the SPSS commands using the Analyze heading. Clicking on the Analyze heading brings up a menu of options for analysis. If you highlight any one of these, a side menu of options is displayed. Highlighting and clicking on one of these suboptions displays a dialog box. The dialog box provides choices that are available in SPSS for the selected statistical test. Figure 8.3 shows the SPSS Frequency dialog box.

In providing instructions for using SPSS commands, we include on the first line of instructions the two or three steps required to get to the first dialog box. These steps are separated by periods (...). Directions for selecting and transferring variables are given next. A √ is used to indicate commands to select. When a new dialog box must

FIGURE 8.2. SPSS DATA EDITOR SCREEN.

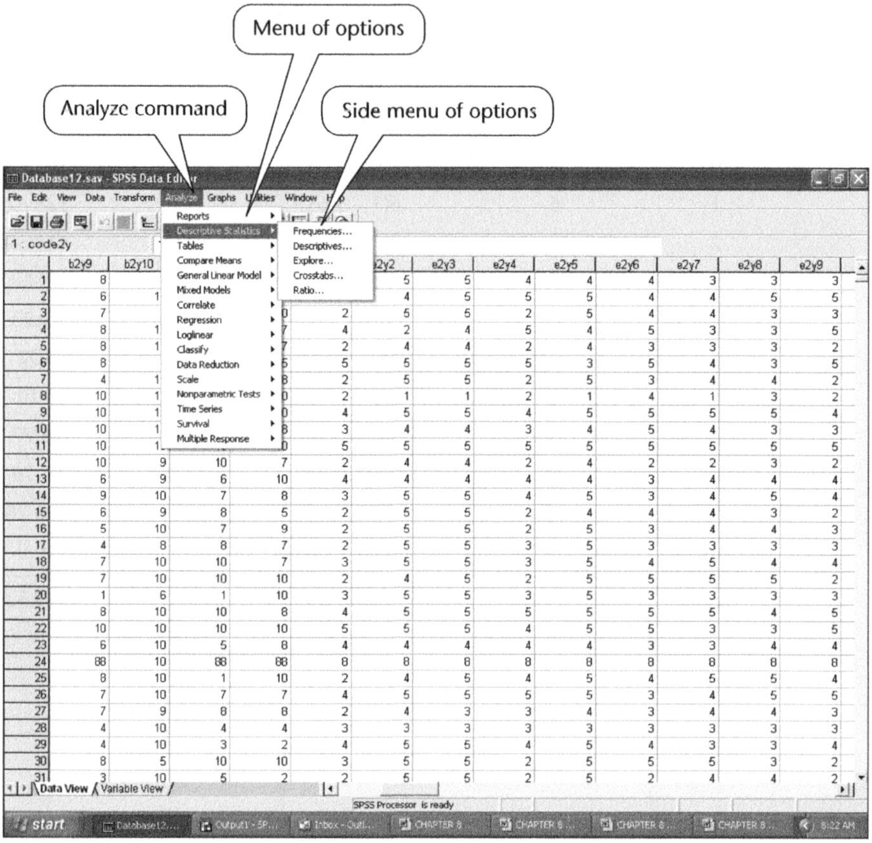

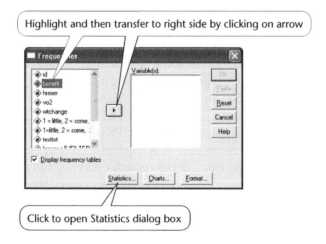

FIGURE 8.3. SPSS DIALOG BOX FOR FREQUENCY.

Highlight and then transfer to right side by clicking on arrow

Click to open Statistics dialog box

be opened to select additional options, the new dialog box is indicated by "(dialog box)" immediately following the commands. Commands are indented and placed under the dialog box in which they appear. Below we give the SPSS commands for calculating the measures of central tendency and dispersion for a set of scores. These commands highlight the information presented regarding the format that we are using for the SPSS instructions. These commands also produced the output in Tables 8.1 and 8.3.

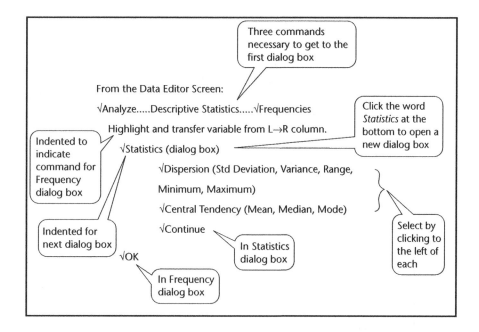

TABLE 8.3. SPSS PRINTOUT OF MEASURES OF CENTRAL TENDENCY AND DISPERSION.

Statistics		
BENEFIT		
N	Valid	100
	Missing	0
Mean		5.6300
Median		6.0000
Mode		9.00
Std. Deviation		3.04065
Variance		9.24556
Range		10.00
Minimum		.00
Maximum		10.00

Recode Negatively Worded Items Using SPSS. When a scale has negatively worded items, it is necessary to reverse score these items before conducting statistical tests. In scale development, total scores are computed based on the idea that a higher score on the scale corresponds to a higher level (more) of the variable being measured. As you know, items on a scale may be worded either positively or negatively. Recall that if an item is positively worded, agreement with the statement represents a higher level of the variable being measured. When an item is negatively worded, agreement with the statement represents a lower level of the variable being measured. There are several methods to accomplish the task of reverse scoring negatively worded items; the method using the SPSS Recode procedure is described here. Be very careful when recoding data. Most statisticians advise students never to permanently change the original data (that is, always maintain the original data file as is). Therefore, we have recommended recoding variables into *new* variables, as shown in the following discussion.

In Chapter Two, we presented the Rosenberg Self-Esteem Scale and noted that five of the ten items are negatively worded: items 3, 5, 8, 9, and 10. That is, strong agreement with these items indicates a low level of self-esteem. In contrast, strong agreement with items 1, 2, 4, 6, and 7 is consistent with a high level of self-esteem. The response options for each item are 1 = *strongly disagree*, 2 = *disagree*, 3 = *agree*, and 4 = *strongly agree*. If we wanted to reverse score the negatively worded items, we would use the SPSS commands that follow.

To reverse score negatively worded items:

From the SPSS Data Editor Screen:

√Transform. . . .Recode. . . .√Into Different Variables

    Highlight and transfer the first item (e.g. Item3) from L column→Input Variable→Output Variable

    In the Output Variable Name box, type a new variable name (e.g. Item3r)

    √Change

    √Old and New Values (dialog box)

        In the Old Value box type in the original value

        In the New Value box type in the recoded value

        √Add

        √Continue

    Repeat sequence for each item to be recoded.

        √Continue

√OK

Using these commands, we can reverse score items 3, 5, 8, 9, and 10 on the Rosenberg Self-Esteem Scale. For each of these items, an original response of "1" is given the new value of "4," a "2" is recoded as a "3," a "3" is recoded as a "2," and a "4" is recoded as a "1." We might label these new variables as Item3r, Item5r, Item8r, Item9r, and Item10r. The *r* denotes that the item has been reversed scored, making a higher number consistent with a higher level of the attribute, in this case, self-esteem. These new variables are automatically added to SPSS database and will appear in the variable list.

Compute Total Scale Scores Using SPSS. Though individual item responses may be of interest, we normally use the individual item responses from a multi-item scale to compute a total score that is intended to represent the level of the variable that is present for an individual. Thus, instead of considering each item individually, we consider the responses to items in a cumulative fashion in order to estimate the level of the variable that is present. The most common approach to creating a total score based on a multi-item scale is to simply take the sum of the item responses. Before calculating a total score, remember to recode any negatively worded items. Follow these commands to create a total scale score.

For the Rosenberg Self-Esteem Scale, the Numeric Expressions box would contain the following expression:

$$\text{Item1} + \text{Item2} + \text{Item3r} + \text{Item4} + \text{Item5r} +$$
$$\text{Item6} + \text{Item7} + \text{Item8r} + \text{Item9r} + \text{Item10r}$$

To compute a total score:

From the SPSS Data Editor Screen:

√Transform. . . .√Compute

    In the Target Variable box, type in new variable name (e.g. esteem)

    Highlight and transfer the first item (e.g. Item1) from L column→Numeric Expressions box

    Enter + sign

    Highlight and transfer the remaining items from L column→Numeric Expressions separating each by a + sign.

√OK

The procedure will create a new variable (e.g., "esteem"), which is the sum of the responses of participants to each of the items on the scale. So if a person gave the following responses to the 10-item scale, he or she would receive a total score of 34 as shown below.

Item	Original Responses	Responses with Recoded Items
1	3	3
2	3	3
3*	2	3
4	4	4
5*	1	4
6	4	4
7	3	3
8*	2	3
9*	2	3
10*	1	4
Total Scale Score		34

* Reversed scored items

The new variable (e.g., "esteem") will be added to the SPSS database and will appear on the variable list.

Review of Correlation

A correlation coefficient provides a measure of the association between variables. We are all familiar with the concept of correlation. It is evident in statements such as, "The risk of skin cancer increases with the amount of sun exposure," "Tobacco use is associated with a higher risk of lung cancer," and, "Unprotected sex increases one's chances of getting HIV." Correlation analysis provides a means of expressing the strength, sign, and significance of these and other associations. The most common type of correlation coefficient is the Pearson product moment correlation coefficient. This is a bivariate correlation, because it examines the correlation between two variables. There are other types of correlations, such as Spearman's rho and multiple correlation, that examine the relationships among more than two variables or a set of variables. The Pearson correlation provides a measure of the strength and sign of the linear relationship between two continuous variables. The relationship between two continuous variables can be presented graphically, as shown in Figures 8.4 and 8.5. In these scatterplots, the values for one variable are plotted along the x-axis and the values for the other are plotted on the y-axis. Figure 8.4 shows the scatterplot for hours of exercise and oxygen consumption (VO_2 ml/kg/min) for the 100 participants enrolled in our healthy lifestyle study. In this hypothetical example, participants were asked how many hours per week they spent participating in aerobic activities. Oxygen consumption (VO_2) was obtained for each person by having each complete a treadmill test. VO_2 is a measure of the amount of oxygen a person consumes per kilogram of body weight per minute. People who are physically fit consume more oxygen per minute during aerobic testing than do those who lead sedentary lifestyles. The scores for each person on both variables are plotted on the scatterplot. Participant A, for example, reported no aerobic activity and had a VO_2 of 30; participant B reported twenty-five hours of aerobic activity per week and had a VO_2 of 52. Note that as the number of hours of exercise increases, so does VO_2. The line through the dots, called a regression line, is the best-fitting line though the points on the graph. The slope of the line reflects the strength of the relationship and the orientation of the line reflects its sign (positive or negative association). In Figure 8.4, the line slopes upward to the right, an indication of a positive correlation.

In Figure 8.5, we see a scatterplot indicative of a negative correlation between two variables. In this case, the regression line slopes downward from left to right, indicating that as the scores on one variable go up, the scores on the other go down. Here the variables are number of hours of exercise per week and change in weight or number of pounds gained or lost during a six-month period of time. The scatterplot shows that the more the person exercises, the less weight he or she gains.

Scatterplots can be used to show the sign of the relationship between two variables. However, the strength of the relationship is best represented by a numerical value often referred to as a correlation coefficient. The most commonly used coefficient is the Pearson product moment. This value is computed using the following formula. In this formula, the Pearson correlation coefficient is represented by the symbol r_{xy}. The subscripts x and y are generally used to denote the two variables.

Equation 8.3

$$r_{xy} = \frac{\Sigma(X - \overline{X})(Y - \overline{Y})}{(N - 1)\, s_x\, s_y}$$

where

r_{xy} = the correlation between the variables X and Y,
Σ = sigma, which indicates to sum what follows
X = the value of the X variable,
$\overline{X}$ = the mean score on the X variable,
Y = the value of the Y variable,
$\overline{Y}$ = the mean score on the Y variable,

FIGURE 8.4. RELATIONSHIP BETWEEN NUMBER OF HOURS EXERCISED AND VO₂ FOR 100 PARTICIPANTS.

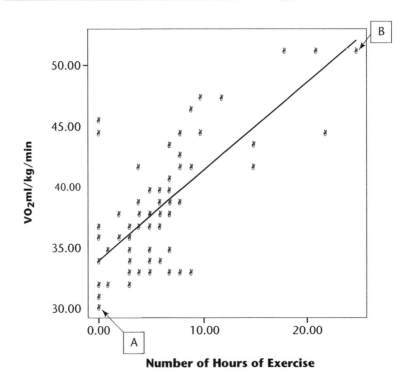

N = the number of observations,

s_x = the standard deviation of the X variable, and

s_y = the standard deviation of the Y variable.

To show the calculation of a correlation, in Table 8.4 we present the responses of ten participants in the exercise study for number of hours of exercise (variable X) and their VO₂s (variable Y). Using the formula given above, we first calculate the deviation from the mean for each of the X and Y scores. We then multiply together each person's x and y deviation values and sum the results for the ten participants. This sum is divided by 9 times the product of the standard deviations for the two distributions (X and Y). The results are shown below.

$$r_{xy} = \frac{305}{(10-1)(7.52)(6.32)}.$$

$$r_{xy} = \frac{305}{427.7} = .713.$$

FIGURE 8.5. RELATIONSHIP BETWEEN NUMBER OF HOURS EXERCISED AND CHANGE IN WEIGHT FOR 100 PARTICIPANTS.

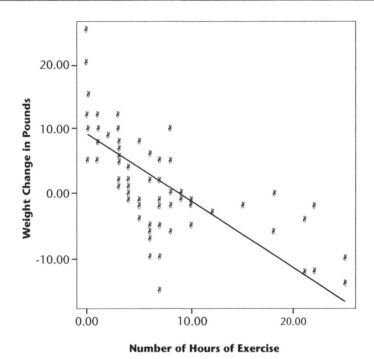

Number of Hours of Exercise

TABLE 8.4. CALCULATION OF THE CORRELATION COEFFICIENT FOR THE ASSOCIATION BETWEEN EXERCISE AND OXYGEN CONSUMPTION.

Person ID	Number of Hours of Exercise	VO₂		
1	0	37	(−10)(−3)	30
2	4	33	(−6)(−7)	42
3	5	35	(−5)(−5)	25
4	6	38	(−4)(−2)	8
5	8	32	(−2)(−8)	16
6	10	45	(.0)(5)	0
7	10	46	(0)(6)	0
8	12	42	(2)(2)	4
9	20	40	(10)(0)	0
10	25	52	(15)(12)	180
Sum				305

At the bottom of the page, we give the SPSS commands for calculating a correlation between two variables.

By convention, Y is the perceived dependent variable, or the presumed outcome, and X is the independent variable, or the presumed cause. In our example, we give the correlation between hours of exercise and VO_2 for the participants in the healthy eating study. In this study, hours of exercise is the independent variable because it logically precedes an increase in VO_2. The value of the correlation computed using SPSS is .753. This value is slightly different from that obtained from our calculations above (.713). Recall that we used a subsample of 10 participants for our calculations, whereas we included all 100 participants in the SPSS calculations.

Interpretation of the Correlation Coefficient

The value of the Pearson correlation coefficient r_{xy} ranges from -1 to $+1$. A perfect negative correlation is represented by -1 and a perfect positive correlation by $+1$. For perfect correlation to exist, every unit increase in the X variable must be matched by a unit increase in the Y variable. The closer the value of r_{xy} is to ± 1, the stronger the correlation is between the two variables. A value of 0 indicates that no relationship exists between the variables. For example, numbers selected at random for the two distributions would be expected to have no association. The correlation between exercise and VO_2 is .753, indicating a strong positive correlation (see Table 8.5). The correlation between number of exercise hours and weight change is $-.671$, indicating a moderately strong negative correlation. Negative correlations occur when scores that are high on one variable correspond to scores that are low on the other variable and vice versa. Students often confuse the strength of the correlation with the sign (+ or −) of the correlation. It is important to remember that the further the value is from 0, the stronger the correlation is, regardless of the sign (Figure 8.6). Thus, the correlation coefficients of $-.25$ and $+.25$ are equivalent in strength but opposite in sign.

To compute a correlation between two variables:

From the Data Entry Screen:

√Analyze. . . .Correlate. . . .√Bivariate correlations

  Highlight and transfer **Y** variable from L→R column

  Highlight and transfer **X** variable from L→R column

  √OK

TABLE 8.5. CORRELATION MATRIX SHOWING RELATIONSHIPS AMONG BENEFIT RATINGS, HOURS OF EXERCISE, VO₂, AND WEIGHT CHANGE.

Correlations

		Benefits	Hours Exercised	VO$_2$	Weight Change
Benefits	Pearson Correlation	1	.632[a]	.492[a]	−.603[a]
	Sig. (2-tailed)		.000	.000	.000
	N	100	100	100	100
Hours Exercised	Pearson Correlation	.632[a]	1	.753[a]	−.671[a]
	Sig. (2-tailed)	.000		.000	.000
	N	100	100	100	100
VO$_2$	Pearson Correlation	.492[a]	.753[a]	1	−.512[a]
	Sig. (2-tailed)	.000	.000		.000
	N	100	100	100	100
Weight Change	Pearson Correlation	−.603[a]	−.671[a]	−.512[a]	1
	Sig. (2-tailed)	.000	.000	.000	
	N	100	100	100	100

1. Correlation coefficient

2. Significance level

3. Number in sample

Diagonal

[a] Correlation is significant at the 0.01 level (2-tailed).

FIGURE 8.6. RANGE AND SIGN OF CORRELATION COEFFICIENTS.

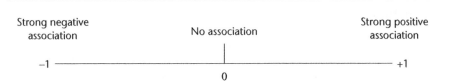

Strong negative association   No association   Strong positive association

−1 ——————————————————————— +1

0

Correlation Matrix

Correlations for a set of variables can be displayed in a correlation matrix, such as the one shown in Table 8.5. The correlation matrix shows the strength, sign, and significance of the relationship between each variable and every other variable. The first number given in each cell of the matrix is the correlation coefficient (1). Table 8.5 presents correlations among the variables discussed earlier: benefit of an exercise program, number of hours of exercise per week, VO_2, and weight change. The correlation between benefit and number of hours of exercise is .632, suggesting a moderately strong positive relationship, whereas the correlation between number of hours of exercise and VO_2 is .753, indicating a strong positive relationship. Note that each relationship between variables is given twice, once above the diagonal and once below. In other words, the correlation table is symmetric, because, for example, the correlation between variable X and variable Y is also equal to the correlation between variable Y and variable X. The order in which the variables are paired does not affect the correlation between them. In reports, researchers generally give only the upper or lower diagonal. The 1's along the diagonal represent the correlation of each variable with itself.

The correlation matrix also gives the p values for statistical significance, which are the second number in each cell (2). The correlation coefficient is a descriptive statistic that provides an indication of the strength and sign of a relationship between two variables. This relationship can be tested using a statistical test. The null hypothesis tested is that no relationship exists between two variables, and the alternative hypothesis is that the relationship does exist. If one is calculating the correlation by hand, as we did in Table 8.4, a statistical table can be used to determine whether the value of the coefficient is significant at the .05 level or the .10 level for a specific sample size. When SPSS is used to calculate correlations, the p value is included in the output. We can see in the correlation matrix that all correlations are significant at the .05 level, meaning that the values of the correlations would occur by chance fewer than 5 out of 100 times when the null hypothesis of no relationship is true. The third number in each cell (3) gives the number of observations used in the calculation of each correlation. In Table 8.5, we see that all 100 observations were used for the calculation of each correlation. If data were missing on one or more participants on a variable, a number less than 100 would appear in the appropriate cell.

Correlation Issues

Causality. There are a few points to remember about correlation. First, correlation does not imply causality even though causation can imply correlation. It is impossible to tell the direction or nature of causation with just the correlation between two variables. For example, Figure 8.7 displays five of many possible scenarios of causation (James, Mulaik, & Brett, 1982). In scenerio a, X is shown as a cause of Y, whereas in

FIGURE 8.7. POSSIBLE CAUSAL RELATIONSHIPS
BETWEEN TWO VARIABLES.

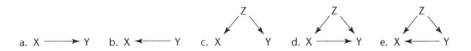

Source: Permission from Stanley A. Mulaik (personal communication, 2005).

scenario b, Y is a cause of X. In the third situation (c), Z is the cause of both X and Y, which are not directly related to each other. In the final two situations (d and e), X and Y are related to each other and also to Z. Knowing only the correlation between two variables cannot help you determine which of these or other scenerios is possible. A more advanced analytic technique known as structural equation modeling (SEM) examines the correlations among many variables to test causal relations. However, SEM has its limits and to show causality, the researcher would need to conduct a controlled experiment to determine the direction of causality. The correlation coefficient does tell us how things are related (descriptive information) and gives us predictive capabilities (if we know the score on one variable, we can predict the score on the other). When we square the correlation coefficient, the result tells us to what extent the variance in one variable explains the variance in the other.

Sample Size. In terms of the statistical significance of the correlation coefficient, the larger the sample size, the more likely it is for the value of r_{xy} to be statistically significant. A correlation of .10 would not be statistically significant for a sample size of 20, but would be significant for a sample size of 1,500. A simple rule of thumb for determining the significance of a correlation coefficient is to compute

$$\frac{2}{\sqrt{N-3}},$$

where N is the sample size (Mulaik, 1972). If the magnitude of the correlation (ignoring its sign) is bigger than this quantity, the correlation is significantly different from zero. So for a sample size of twenty, the correlation would need to be at least .50 to be statistically significant as shown below:

$$\frac{2}{\sqrt{20-3}} = \frac{2}{\sqrt{17}} = \frac{2}{4} = .5.$$

In the case of correlations, statistical significance does not say much about practical significance. With a fairly large sample size, we might find that the correlation between drinking coffee and skin cancer is .09. However, with such a small correlation, it is unlikely that health professionals would tell people to give up coffee to avoid skin cancer or would include this information in a pamphlet on skin protection.

Group Differences. In research, we might find that the association between two variables differs for groups. This difference in association might be apparent when the correlations are analyzed separately for each group. However, when the groups are combined, the differences might be obscured. For example, if we analyzed them separately, we might find a strong positive correlation between eating chocolate and weight gain for women and a small negative correlation for men. When data from both men and women are analyzed together, we might find no relationship between eating chocolate and weight gain for the total sample, leading to a conclusion that is not true for either group. Likewise, we can have negative (or positive) correlations between two variables in two groups, but get a near zero or slightly positive (or negative) correlation when the groups are combined. In these cases, the correlations may be due not to individual sources of variation but to sources introduced by group membership, and the group effect cancels the relationship due to individual sources.

Restriction of Range. Researchers should also be aware of the possibility of a situation known as restriction of range. If the range of one or both scores involved in a correlation is restricted or reduced, the correlation may be different from a similar correlation based on an unrestricted range of scores. Correlations in the restricted sample may be reduced, showing no correlation, when there is a correlation in the unrestricted population. Likewise, nonzero correlations between variables may occur in restricted populations when there is no correlation between the variables in an unrestricted population. In Figure 8.8, we limit our analysis for our healthy lifestyle study to men and women who report that they exercise less than five hours per week. With this restricted group of participants, we see that the correlation between number of hours of exercise and VO_2 is .224 and is not statistically significant. This correlation leads to the conclusion that there is no association between number of hours of exercise and VO_2. However, if we include people in the higher range, who exercised more hours and had higher VO_2 levels, as shown earlier in Figure 8.4, a distinct positive correlation exists. Thus, restricting the range of variables may lead to inaccurate conclusions about the association between variables.

Variance

Earlier, we defined variance for a single frequency distribution. We said it was the average squared distance from the mean. We can also calculate the percentage of variance in one distribution that is shared with another distribution. By squaring the

FIGURE 8.8. RELATIONSHIP BETWEEN NUMBER OF HOURS EXERCISED AND VO$_2$ FOR THOSE WHO EXERCISE FEWER THAN FIVE HOURS PER WEEK.

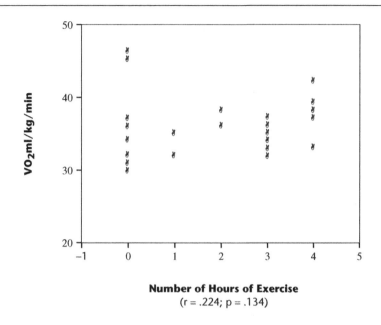

Number of Hours of Exercise
(r = .224; p = .134)

correlation coefficient, r_{xy}, we find the proportion of variance in one variable accounted for by its relationship with the other variable.

The percentage of shared variance can be represented using Venn diagrams, as shown in Figures 8.9 and 8.10. In Figure 8.9, each circle represents 100 percent of the variance in one variable. The circle on the left might represent the total amount of variance for number of hours of exercise, and the circle on the right might represent the total amount of variance for VO$_2$ scores.

We saw earlier that the correlation coefficient for the relationship between these two variables was .753. This finding indicates that the two variables share a large portion of variance. Figure 8.10 depicts the shared variance, using two intersecting circles. The area of overlap between the circles denotes the proportion of shared variance. We can calculate the amount of shared variance by squaring the correlation coefficient. Squaring r_{xy} yields a decimal number that can be converted to a percentage by multiplying it by 100. The value obtained from squaring the correlation coefficient is referred to as the coefficient of determination and can be interpreted as the proportion of shared variance between two variables. Shared variance is usually presented as a percentage ranging from 0 to 100 percent. In the computation below, we show the calculation of the percent of shared variance for number of hours of exercise and VO$_2$.

FIGURE 8.9. VENN DIAGRAM SHOWING VARIANCE FOR TWO SEPARATE VARIABLES.

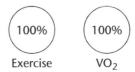

Exercise   VO$_2$

Equation 8.4

$$r_{xy}^2 \times 100 = \text{percent of shared variance}$$
$$.753^2 \times 100 = 57\%.$$

We can then say that 57 percent of the variance in VO$_2$ is shared with number of hours of exercise or that 57 percent of VO$_2$ is explained by exercise.

If two variables are not associated at all, then $r_{xy} = 0$ and r_{xy}^2 will be .00 (or 0 percent). That is, there is no variance that the two variables share. Conversely, when two variables are perfectly correlated, $r_{xy} = 1$ and $r_{xy}^2 = 1.0$ (or 100 percent). Thus, 100 percent of the variance in the first variable is explained by the second variable and vice versa.

Reporting Results of Correlation Analysis

It might be helpful to select a few correlations for interpretation. We will begin with the correlation between number of hours of exercise and VO$_2$. The correlation coefficient r_{xy} is .75 and $p < .001$. These results indicate that the variables are positively correlated. That is, as the number of hours a person exercises increases, so does that person's VO$_2$. A correlation coefficient value of .75 is fairly strong. This value indicates that 57 percent of the variance in VO$_2$ is explained by hours of exercise and vice versa. The p value $< .001$ indicates that the relationship is statistically significant. That is, given a null hypothesis stating that $p = 0$, the probability of obtaining a correlation of the given magnitude (.753) purely by chance is estimated to be less than 1 percent.

As a second example, the correlation between number of hours of exercise and weight change is $r_{xy} = -.67$ and the p value is $< .001$. The association is strong and negative as hours of exercise increase weight gain decreases. We can say that 45 percent of the variance in number of pounds gained or lost is explained by the number of hours of exercise. Given a null hypothesis stating that $p = 0$, the probability of obtaining a correlation of the given magnitude (.671) purely by chance is estimated to be less than 1 percent.

FIGURE 8.10. VENN DIAGRAM SHOWING THE SHARED VARIANCE BETWEEN TWO VARIABLES.

Exercise   VO$_2$

Analysis of Variance

Definition and Use

Although much of reliability and validity analysis is based on correlations, some assessments require an understanding of statistics to compare group means. In this section, we describe ANOVA, which is a set of analytic procedures used to compare means for two or more groups of participants. ANOVA procedures focus on comparing two variance estimates. One estimate is based on differences between group means and reflects variance due to group differences plus error. The second estimate is based on the variability among scores within a group; this estimate is considered to be random or error variance. We will limit our discussion to the one-way ANOVA, which has only one independent variable. The independent t test is a special case of one-way ANOVA and can be used in its place when there are only two groups under consideration. We present the one-way ANOVA because it is a more general approach than the t test.

ANOVA is used to test statistical hypotheses that propose differences between group means. Suppose that the researcher conducting the healthy lifestyle study is interested in knowing whether or not there is a difference in benefit ratings based on the number of hours a person exercises each week. Based on the health belief model, the researcher hypothesizes that participants who spend more time exercising each week will rate the benefit of exercise higher. The researcher divides the sample into three groups, based on their reported hours of weekly exercise. Participants in group 1 are those who exercise three or fewer hours per week, those in group 2 exercise between four and seven hours per week, and those in group 3 exercise more than seven hours per week. The researcher labels the groups as follows: 1 = *a little,* 2 = *some,* and 3 = *a great deal.* To conduct the ANOVA, mean scores for the dependent variable (in this case, benefit ratings) for each exercise group are computed. Recall that the benefit of exercise was rated on a eleven-point scale from *no benefit at all* (0) to a *great deal of benefit* (10), and higher scores are associated with greater perceived benefit of exercise. The means of the benefit ratings for each group are compared to one another. The group variable (in this case, exercise group) is the independent variable.

According to the health belief model, group 3 would be expected to rate the benefit of exercise the highest, followed by group 2 and then group 1.

SPSS Commands for a One-Way ANOVA

The computation for ANOVA can be found in statistical texts such as Kleinbaum, Kupper, Muller, and Nizam (1997). Here we only show the SPSS commands. It is important to remember that the ANOVA procedure requires that the independent variable be categorical (that is, nominal or ordinal) and that the dependent variable be continuous (that is, interval or ratio).

Interpreting a One-Way ANOVA

As noted previously, an ANOVA tests the difference between (or among) group means. The statistic computed and evaluated to determine whether differences exist is the F test. An F test that is statistically significant indicates that there is a better-than-chance difference between the mean scores of at least two of the groups. If there are more than two groups and the overall F test is statistically significant, a follow-up (or post hoc) test is conducted to identify the specific group differences. Though a number of post hoc test options exist, the choice of a particular test should be based on the characteristics of the distributions under consideration. For simplicity, Tukey's post hoc test is presented.

To conduct a one-way ANOVA:

From the Data Editor Screen:

√Analyze. . . .Compare Means. . . .√One-Way ANOVA

    Highlight and transfer **X** variable into the Factor box

    Highlight and transfer **Y** variable into the Dependent List box

        √Options (dialog box)

            √Descriptive

            √Homogeneity of Variance Test

        √Continue

        √Post-Hoc (dialog box)

        √Tukey

            √Continue

    √OK

Table 8.6 presents the first table from the SPSS output. This table, labeled Descriptives, provides group and overall descriptive statistics for the dependent variable (in this case, benefit rating). From a strictly descriptive perspective, the means of the three groups appear to be different. In particular, the mean benefit rating for group 1 is 3.14, that for group 2 is 6.22, and that for group 3 is 8.07.

Table 8.7, labeled Test of Homogeneity of Variances, provides the results of Levene's test, which can be used to determine whether the homogeneity-of-variance assumption is tenable. The null hypothesis for this test is that the variances across the groups are equal. In this situation we want to retain the null hypothesis; therefore, we are looking for a p value >.05. Table 8.7 shows that the Levene statistic of .769 is not statistically significant ($p = .466$), and we can accept the null hypothesis that the variances are equal.

TABLE 8.6 SPSS PRINTOUT USING THE ONE-WAY ANOVA DESCRIPTIVE COMMAND.

Mean scores for benefit (dependent variable) by exercise group

Descriptives

BENEFIT

	N	Mean	Std. Deviation	Std. Error	95% Confidence Interval for Mean Lower Bound	95% Confidence Interval for Mean Upper Bound	Minimum	Maximum
1.00	36	3.1389	2.33180	.38863	2.3499	3.9279	.00	9.00
2.00	36	6.2222	2.35568	.39261	5.4252	7.0193	2.00	10.00
3.00	28	8.0714	2.17611	.41125	7.2276	8.9152	2.00	10.00
Total	100	5.6300	3.04065	.30407	5.0267	6.2333	.00	10.00

Exercise group (independent variable)

TABLE 8.7. SPSS PRINTOUT FOR TEST OF HOMOGENEITY OF VARIANCES.

Test of Homogeneity of Variances

BENEFIT

Levene Statistic	df1	df2	Sig.
.769	2	97	.466

Look for a p value >.05

Table 8.8, labeled ANOVA, gives the results of the one-way ANOVA test. Remember, the F test in this case is an omnibus test; that is, the F test provides evidence that there is at least one pairwise difference between the groups under consideration. The p value for the overall F test is in the last column of the table. A $p < .05$ indicates that there is a statistically significant difference between at least two of the groups. In Table 8.8, the F statistic is 38.139 and the p value is $< .001$, indicating that the means for at least two of the groups are statistically different from each other.

Table 8.9, labeled Multiple Comparisons, presents the results of the post hoc comparison (in this example, using Tukey's HSD [honestly significantly different] test). The Multiple Comparisons table provides information for all pairwise comparisons (that is, each group mean is compared to every other group mean). If the p value for any row in this table were less than the designated value (for example, .05), the difference between the means for the two groups under consideration would be considered a statistically significant difference (or a better-than-chance difference). As noted in Table 8.9, the mean differences between all comparisons are statistically significant. To find the mean difference, subtract each group listed on the right in the first column from the group listed on the left in this column. So for the first row, subtract 6.222 (the mean of group 2) from 3.1389 (the mean for group 1) to obtain the mean difference

TABLE 8.8. SPSS PRINTOUT OF ANOVA SUMMARY TABLE.

ANOVA

> F ratio: calculated by dividing the mean square between by the mean square within

BENEFIT

	Sum of Squares	df	Mean Square	F	Sig.
Between Groups	402.925	2	201.463	38.139	.000
Within Groups	512.385	97	5.282		
Total	915.310	99			

> Variation is partitioned into variability due to group differences (between) and variability due to individual differences (within) within each group

> Degrees of freedom

> p value associated with the observed F statistic ($p < .05$), indicating a statistically significant result—reject the null that the group means are equal

TABLE 8.9. SPSS PRINTOUT SHOWING COMPARISONS AMONG THE GROUPS.

Multiple Comparisons

> p values identify the statistically significant pairwise group differences

Dependent Variable: BENEFIT
Tukey HSD

(I) 1=little, 2=some, 3 = a lot	(J) 1=little, 2=some, 3 = a lot	Mean Difference (I-J)	Std. Error	Sig.	95% Confidence Interval	
					Lower Bound	Upper Bound
1.00	2.00	−3.0833*	.54172	.000	−4.3728	−1.7939
	3.00	−4.9325*	.57912	.000	−6.3110	−3.5541
2.00	1.00	3.0833*	.54172	.000	1.7939	4.3728
	3.00	−1.8492*	.57912	.005	−3.2277	−.4708
3.00	1.00	4.9325*	.57912	.000	3.5541	6.3110
	2.00	1.8492*	.57912	.005	.4708	3.2277

> To obtain results in column 2 subtract the mean of the group listed to the right from that listed on the left

*The mean difference is significant at the .05 level.

of −3.0833. By examining the direction of the mean differences as noted in the first column, we see that group 2 (some exercise) and group 3 (a lot of exercise) have higher mean scores than group 1 (little exercise) and that group 3 has a higher mean score than group 2. These results suggest that participants who exercise the most rate the most benefit of exercise. Those who exercise a moderate amount fall somewhere in between.

In summary, then, our researcher can say that there is a difference in perceived benefit of exercise among participants based on the number of hours they exercise each week. Those participants who exercise the most report the most benefit. Those participants who report exercising a moderate amount each week rate the benefit of exercise lower than do those reporting more than seven hours of exercise per week, but higher than do those reporting only a few hours of exercise per week.

Summary

In this chapter, we have presented a review of some statistical concepts that are important to understand in order to conduct assessments for reliability and validity of scales. Many of the tests used to evaluate reliability and validity are based on correlation. Some validity assessments also require the use of analysis of variance. The information presented in this chapter should be sufficient to understand the analyses presented in later chapters. However, students who wish to read more about correlation and about ANOVA and other statistical tests are referred to the texts by Kleinbaum, Kupper, Muller, and Nizam (1997), Norman and Streiner (2000), and Tabachnick and Fidell (2001). Students who wish to read more about SPSS can consult the SPSS manual or a how-to text such as that by Cronk (1999).

CHAPTER NINE

FUNDAMENTALS OF RELIABILITY

LEARNING OBJECTIVES

At the end of this chapter, the student should be able to

1. Understand the relationship between random error and reliability.
2. Define the terms *observed score, true score,* and *error score.*
3. Define the term *reliability.*
4. Describe the theoretical equation representing the relationship among the observed, true, and error scores.
5. Use the theoretical equation to compute observed-score, true-score, and error-score variance.
6. Use the theoretical equation to compute the reliability coefficient.
7. Understand the relationship between the observed score and true score and the reliability coefficient.
8. State the relationship between the correlation of two parallel tests and reliability.
9. Use the reliability coefficient to determine the proportion of observed-score variance due to true-score and error-score variance.
10. Use the reliability coefficient to determine the reliability index.

When respondents in a research study answer questions about health behaviors, there is always a possibility of error. One respondent might misread an item about exercise; another might overestimate the amount of exercise he or she does each week. Small or occasional errors are not likely to have a great effect on a person's over-all score. For example, the total score for a respondent who enters a 3 instead of a 2 for one item on a twenty-item scale will be inflated by one point. If the respondent an-swers the same items without error a week later, under the same conditions, the total score will differ by only one point. Conversely, if testing conditions are poor, the items ambiguous, and the format of the scale confusing, a respondent may have difficulty answering the items. If asked to answer the same items again, the respondent may se-lect different answers. A difference in answers that cannot be attributed to actual change in knowledge, attitudes, opinions, or behavior is likely due to error.

The term *reliability* refers to consistency, repeatability, and reproducibility. Instruments that provide consistent scores are said to be reliable, or dependable. An instrument is reliable to the extent that it can be demonstrated that on repeated use of the instrument, the scores are not affected by random errors. As random error increases, so does the variability of scores. And as the variability of scores increases due to error, the reproducibility, or consistency, of the scores decreases.

A good way to represent consistency on repeated measures is shown in the histograms in Figures 9.1 and 9.2. Suppose the first histogram is a depiction of the scores a stu-dent, Josh, receives on 100 attempts at taking the same research methods test. Assume that each of his attempts is independent of all the others, that is, that each attempt is not influenced by previous attempts (practice effect). Notice the variability or dispersion in his scores for these attempts. Compare this variability to that in the second histogram,

FIGURE 9.1. HISTOGRAM OF JOSH'S SCORES ON 100 REPEATED ATTEMPTS ON A RESEARCH METHODS TEST.

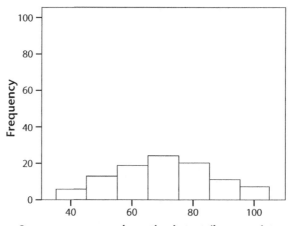

Scores on a research methods test (low consistency)

FIGURE 9.2. HISTOGRAM OF JOSH'S SCORES ON 100 REPEATED ATTEMPTS ON A HEALTH BEHAVIOR THEORY TEST.

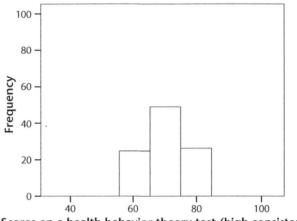

which represents Josh's test-taking attempts on a health behavior theory test taken 100 times. Notice that the scores he receives from the attempts on the theory test are closer to the mean than those on the research methods test. The scores on the theory test are considered more reliable, because on repeated attempts the scores are more consistent and cluster around the mean, indicating the presence of little random error. Given these results, the reliability (or consistency) of scores for the theory test is greater than that for the research methods test. When using a reliable instrument, a researcher anticipates that the score obtained for any one test is a fairly good reflection of the person's "true" score on the instrument.

Classical Test Theory

Observed, True, and Error Scores

The true-score model has been used to address issues related to measurement error. During the past century, this model has evolved to explain the concept of reliability and is called classical test theory (CTT). CTT is based on the idea that there is always a true score associated with an individual's response on an instrument. The true score is the person's *real* level of knowledge, strength of opinion or attitude, or measure of skill or behavior as obtained under ideal conditions. Because no measure is perfect, the actual or observed scores on an instrument are assumed to include some error. The relationships among true, error, and observed scores are expressed in the following equation.

Equation 9.1

Observed score = **T**rue score + **E**rror score,

where the observed score (O) reflects the actual score a respondent obtains on an instrument, the true score (T) reflects the actual level or degree of the attribute possessed by the respondent, and the error score (E) reflects the amount of error present in the observed score at the time of measurement.

Because the true and error scores are latent (that is, unobservable), a set of assumptions is necessary in order to use CTT to understand reliability. The first assumption addresses the mean of the error scores. Because error is random, sometimes inflating a score and sometimes decreasing a score, it is assumed that random errors

---

Definition of Error Score

In the context of CTT, error is not the same as the wrong answer on a test. If one knows the correct answer but selects the wrong answer, a CTT error has occurred. Likewise, if one does not know the correct answer but selects the correct one, a CTT error has occurred. A CTT error occurs when the answer to a test—the opinion, belief, or feeling that is selected—is different from what one would have selected under ideal test conditions.

Definition of Parallel Tests

Parallel tests are tests that have the same mean, variance, and correlations with other tests. They also contain items from the same content domain and are theoretically identical, but they have different items. The Scholastic Aptitude Test (SAT) is a good example of a test with parallel forms. SAT tests are often administered in large rooms. Students sitting next to each other are given different forms of the SAT (Form A or Form B). Although the items on the two forms are different, it is assumed that the content assessed and the characteristics of the items are the same for the two forms.

will cancel out *over multiple tests* so that the sum and mean of the error scores are both 0. A second assumption is that the true and error scores are not correlated, and a third assumption is that the error scores across parallel tests are not correlated.

Assumptions and Characteristics

The following example will help clarify the first assumption, that the sum and mean of error scores are equal to 0. Table 9.1 displays a set of scores for Josh, who takes the same research methods quiz ten times. Assume that each of his attempts is independent of all the others. In addition to the actual scores (observed scores) on the quiz, Table 9.1 presents Josh's true score on the quiz, or the score he would have obtained without errors. In the final column is the error score for each attempt on the quiz, or O–T. There are a few important points to be made about the information in Table 9.1. First, note that when the error scores are summed, they cancel each other out, and the total error score for this set of scores is 0. Thus, sometimes Josh made errors that resulted in an observed score that was higher than his true score, and at other times, he made errors that resulted in an observed score that was lower than his true score. Because errors are assumed to be random, we expect that the number of positive errors will be equal to the number of negative errors and that these will cancel each other out over multiple tests. Thus, both the total error score and the mean error score will equal 0. Second, note that although the mean error score is 0, there is variability, or variance, associated with the error scores.

Table 9.1 also shows that the observed-score mean is equal to the true score. If we assume that the mean error score over multiple tests is 0, then the mean of the

TABLE 9.1. JOSH'S OBSERVED, TRUE, AND ERROR SCORES FOR TEN ATTEMPTS ON A RESEARCH METHODS QUIZ.

Quiz Attempt	Observed Scores	True Scores	Error Scores (O–T)
1	4	3	1
2	2	3	−1
3	5	3	2
4	5	3	2
5	1	3	−2
6	3	3	0
7	3	3	0
8	2	3	−1
9	2	3	−1
10	3	3	0
Mean	3	3	0
Variance	1.78	0	1.78
Standard Deviation	1.33	0	1.33

observed score will always be equal to the true score. Thus, the best estimate of the true score is the mean of the observed scores. Note also that the variance of the observed score is equal to the sum of the variance of the true score plus the variance of the error score. In this example, the variance of the true score is 0. Thus, the variance in the observed score is due completely to error variance. Note also that the standard deviation of the error score is 1.33. Another name for the standard deviation of error scores is the *standard error of measurement.*

When we think of reliability, we think of consistency of scores on repeated use of an instrument for groups of people. Thus, we need to shift our focus from the scores of one person taking a test numerous times to the use of an instrument to measure the knowledge, attitudes, opinions, or behaviors of many people. The assumptions of CTT are the same for a set of scores from different respondents as they are for a set of scores from one respondent: (1) the mean error score for a sample is expected to be 0, (2) true scores are not correlated with error scores, indicating that people who have different ability levels or have different opinions or attitudes are equally likely to make random errors, and (3) the error scores on parallel tests are not correlated with each other.

Table 9.2 presents the true, observed, and error scores on three different research methods tests taken by ten students. The first column of Table 9.2 shows the identification number (ID) for each student; the second column shows the students' true scores (this is a theoretical value whose exact value is never really known); the next three columns show each student's observed scores for the three tests (tests 1 through 3); and the final three columns show error scores for each of the three tests (errors 1 through 3). The error scores were obtained by subtracting the true score from each corresponding observed score. Notice that the mean of each set of observed scores is approximately equal to the mean of the true scores, and that the mean for each set of error score is

TABLE 9.2. DESCRIPTIVE STATISTICS FOR TRUE SCORES, PARALLEL TEST SCORES, AND ERROR SCORES FOR A SAMPLE OF STUDENTS.

ID	True	Test 1	Test 2	Test 3	Error 1	Error 2	Error 3
1	95	100	90	93	+5	-5	-2
2	92	94	100	96	+2	+8	+4
3	90	88	98	86	-2	+8	-4
4	88	78	84	92	-10	-4	+4
5	87	90	84	92	+3	-3	+5
6	82	80	84	75	-2	+2	-7
7	76	82	70	74	+6	-6	-2
8	70	74	72	68	+4	+2	-2
9	65	62	68	69	-3	+3	+4
10	60	60	62	58	0	+2	-2
Mean	80.5	80.8	81.2	80.3	.3	.7	-.2

close to 0, supporting assumption 1. We present a small sample here; however, as the number of respondents increases, the mean of the observed scores will approach the mean of the true scores, and the mean of the error scores will approach 0.

Table 9.3 shows a correlation matrix for the correlations among the true, observed, and error scores presented in Table 9.2. These correlations help clarify the second and third assumptions of CTT—that true scores are not correlated with error scores and errors are not correlated across parallel tests. First, notice the relationships between the true and error scores (1). The correlations, which range from −.009 to .089, are low and for all practical purposes can be considered negligible. This finding suggests that there is no association between students' knowledge of the content of the test and random errors, supporting assumption 2, that there is no relationship between true and error scores. Thus, students who know the content well make about the same number of random errors as those who are not as well informed.

Second, examine the correlation among the error scores of the three parallel tests (2). These correlations range from −.094 to −.205, and although the correlations are

TABLE 9.3. CORRELATIONS AMONG TRUE SCORES, PARALLEL TEST SCORES, AND ERROR SCORES FOR A SAMPLE OF STUDENTS.

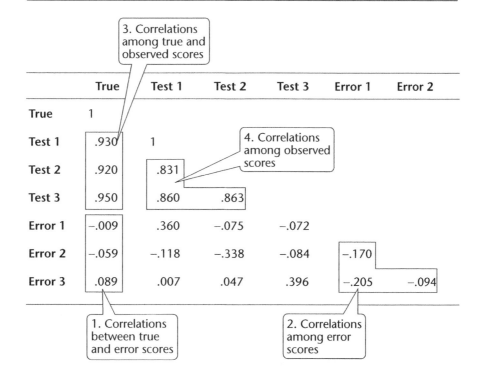

	True	Test 1	Test 2	Test 3	Error 1	Error 2
True	1					
Test 1	.930	1				
Test 2	.920	.831				
Test 3	.950	.860	.863			
Error 1	−.009	.360	−.075	−.072		
Error 2	−.059	−.118	−.338	−.084	−.170	
Error 3	.089	.007	.047	.396	−.205	−.094

3. Correlations among true and observed scores

4. Correlations among observed scores

1. Correlations between true and error scores

2. Correlations among error scores

not 0, as would be expected according to theory, they are close enough to 0 to be considered insignificant. This finding indicates that errors from one test are not associated with errors on another test (assumption 3). In other words, the same respondents are not making the same errors on each test. One person might have had a headache and might have missed several items on the first test, but felt fine for the second test and answered these items correctly. Another person might have done well on the first test and on the second test made mistakes due to pressure to complete the exam quickly because of a pending appointment.

In addition to demonstrating assumptions 2 and 3, Table 9.3 presents correlations showing the relationship between true and observed scores (3) and among the observed scores (4). The correlations between the true and observed scores range from .920 to .950, indicating a fairly high association between the true and observed scores. This means that respondents who really know the content well are also obtaining higher scores on the test, and those who really do not know the content are answering fewer items correctly. The correlations among the observed scores range from .831 to .863. Although these correlations are not as high as those between true and observed scores, the relationships are strong, indicating that students who obtain high scores on one test also tend to score high on the others. We will return to the discussion of the correlations between observed scores in the next section.

Reliability Coefficient

Now that we understand what reliability is, we turn our attention to estimating reliability. To appreciate the interpretation of reliability, it is important to understand the connection between variance and the reliability coefficient. Recall that the term *variance* refers to variability or dispersion in a set of scores. Some variance in observed scores will be due to true differences among respondents, and some will be due to random error. We can depict the relationship as that in Figure 9.3, which shows that the observed-score variance is composed of both true-score and error-score variance.

FIGURE 9.3. RELATIONSHIP AMONG OBSERVED-, TRUE-, AND ERROR-SCORE VARIANCE.

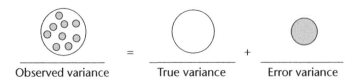

Observed variance = True variance + Error variance

The theoretical equation for this relationship is

Equation 9.2

$$VAR(O) = VAR(T) + VAR(E),$$

where *VAR* refers to variance, and *O*, *T*, and *E* refer to observed, true, and error scores.

A set of scores in which the observed-score variance is made up primarily of true-score variance is more reliable (consistent) than one in which the observed-score variance is made up primarily of error variance. This is because true-score variance will remain unchanged on repeated administrations of an instrument under identical conditions, whereas error-score variance is subject to change. The more error that is reflected in an observed score, the more inconsistent scores will be on repeated administrations of the instrument. Reliability is defined theoretically as the proportion of variance in the observed score that is explained by the true score. This relationship is shown in Equation 9.3.

Equation 9.3

$$r_{ot}^2 = \frac{VAR(T)}{VAR(O)},$$

where

r_{ot}^2 = the reliability coefficient,
$VAR(T)$ = the true-score variance, and
$VAR(O)$ = the observed-score variance.

Using Equation 9.2, we can substitute [*VAR(T)* + *VAR(E)*] for *VAR(O)*.

Equation 9.4

$$r_{ot}^2 = \frac{VAR(T)}{VAR(T) + VAR(E)}.$$

From Equation 9.4, we can show that when the observed-score variance in a test is due entirely to true-score variance, the denominator will equal the numerator and the reliability coefficient will equal 1. Conversely, if the observed-score variance is due entirely to error variance, the reliability coefficient will equal 0. In general, as the proportion of *VAR(T)* increases, r_{ot}^2 approaches 1, and as the proportion of *VAR(E)* increases, r_{ot}^2 approaches 0. The reliability coefficient ranges in value from 0 to 1; coefficients closer to 1 reflect a higher proportion of true-score variance.

A few examples will help demonstrate the relationship among observed-, true-, and error-score variance. If the true-score variance of an instrument is 9, and the error-score variance is 1, then

$$r^2_{ot} = \frac{9}{9+1} = \frac{9}{10} = .90.$$

If the true-score variance of an instrument is 3 and the error-score variance is 12, then

$$r^2_{ot} = \frac{3}{3+12} = \frac{3}{15} = .20.$$

In the first example, 90 percent of the observed-score variance is due to true-score variance, and in the second example, only 20 percent of the observed-score variance is due to true-score variance. The scores obtained from the first instrument are considered more reliable than the scores from the second.

Estimate of Reliability

Equation 9.4 has two unknowns: true-score and error-score variance. To use this equation, we must know the variance of the observed score and the variance of either the true score or the error score. Because we have said that neither the true score nor the error score is known, we must use other means to estimate the proportion of variance in the observed scores that is due to the true scores. One common estimate of the reliability coefficient is the correlation between observed scores on parallel tests. Consider the observed scores in Table 9.3. If all the students took the three tests without random error, the students' observed scores on the parallel tests would equal their true scores. In this case, the correlation between any two parallel tests would be 1, a perfect correlation. The extent to which the value of the correlation coefficient is less than perfect provides an indication of the amount of error variance that is present. Because random error is always present, it is more likely that the correlation between two parallel tests will be less than 1. Notice among the observed scores in Table 9.3 that the correlations between parallel tests are less than 1, ranging from .831 to .863. According to CTT, the proportion of true-score variance in an instrument is equal to the correlation between two parallel tests. The amount of error present is the difference between a perfect correlation coefficient (1.0), which assumes no error, and the value of the correlation for the parallel tests.

For example, in Table 9.3, the correlation between Test 1 and Test 2 is .83. The proportion of true-score variance for either test is estimated to be 83 percent (.83 × 100%), and the proportion of error score variance is

Equation 9.5

$$VAR(E) = 1 - r_{ot}^2, \text{ so}$$
$$.17 = 1 - .83, \text{ and}$$
$$.17 \times 100 = 17\%.$$

We can say that 83 percent of the variance in the observed score is due to the true-score variance, and 17 percent is due to error-score variance. For two parallel tests, the relationship between the correlation coefficient and the reliability coefficient is shown in Equation 9.6:

Equation 9.6

$$r_{x1x2} = r_{ot}^2,$$

where

r_{x1x2} = the correlation between parallel tests, and
r_{ot}^2 = the reliability coefficient, or proportion of variance, in the observed score explained by the true score.

The astute student will note that a correlation coefficient obtained from empirical data (observed scores) is interpreted as a proportion of true-score variance in a theoretical equation. This is an important concept that is often confusing to students.

Calculation of Variance Due to the True Score

If we know the standard deviation or the variance of the observed scores and the reliability coefficient, we can calculate the proportion of variance due to true and error scores. Equation 9.3 can be rewritten as follows:

Equation 9.7

$$VAR(T) = r_{ot}^2 \times VAR(O).$$

Expressed in words, the variance of the true score [*VAR(T)*] is equal to the reliability coefficient multiplied by the variance of the observed score [*VAR(O)*].

In the above example, the correlation between Test 1 and Test 2 is .83. If the variance of test 1 is 165, then

$$.83 \times 165 = 137,$$

where 137 is the variance of the true scores. To find the amount of variance due to error, we subtract the true-score variance from the observed-score variance as follows:

$$165 - 137 = 28,$$

where 28 is the variance of the error scores.

Here is another example. Suppose a group of respondents complete two different versions of a self-esteem scale. The value of the correlation coefficient for the association between the two measures is .81. Using the correlation as an estimate of reliability of either of the two scales, we can say that 81 percent of the observed-score variance is attributable to true-score variance for this group. Subtracting .81 from 1.0, we can show that .19 (or 19 percent) of the observed-score variance is due to error-score variance. If the standard deviation of the observed scores is 4, then

$$VAR(O) = 4^2 = 16,$$
$$VAR(T) = .81 \times 16 = 12.96 \text{ (Equation 9.7), and}$$
$$VAR(E) = 16 - 12.96 = 3.04 \text{ (Equation 9.4).}$$

Calculation of the Reliability Index

We can determine the correlation between the observed score and the true score by taking the square root of the reliability coefficient. Thus:

Equation 9.8

$$r_{ot} = \sqrt{r_{ot}^2},$$

where

r_{ot} = the correlation between observed score and true score.

This value is also referred to as the reliability index.

Summary

In this chapter, we have discussed classical test theory and its relationship with reliability. The term *reliability* refers to consistency, repeatability, and reproducibility. In classical test theory, reliability is defined as the percentage of observed-score variance explained by the true-score variance. Reliability is the part of the variance that is due to true scores and not to error scores. Because true-score variance is never known, we use empirical estimates of reliability to estimate the proportion of observed-score variance explained by the true score. In Chapter Ten, we will discuss these estimates of reliability, which are based on (1) consistency between scores on alternate or parallel tests, (2) consistency of scores over time (stability or test-retest reliability), (3) consistency among items on a scale, and (4) consistency of scores obtained by the same observer in the course of more than one observation or scores obtained by more than one observer. Students who are interested in reading more about classical test theory should read Crocker and Algina (1986), Pedhazur and Schmelkin (1991), or Nunnally and Bernstein (1994).

CHAPTER TEN

RELIABILITY ASSESSMENT
AND ITEM ANALYSIS

LEARNING OBJECTIVES

At the end of this chapter, the student should be able to

1. Describe the characteristics of reliability.
2. Describe the procedures for assessing reliability.
3. State advantages and disadvantages of each type of reliability.
4. Make adjustments in scales to improve reliability.
5. Use SPSS to run reliability tests.
6. Interpret SPSS printouts for coefficient alpha reliability.
7. Use an SPSS printout to assess item characteristics.
8. Use SPSS to calculate intrarater reliability.
9. Describe the basic components of generalizability theory.

In Chapter Nine, we learned that reliability is the degree of consistency with which an instrument measures what it is intended to measure. From a classical test theory (CTT) view, reliability is defined as the proportion of the observed-score variance that is explained by the true-score variance. We also learned that we are unlikely to know the true score and therefore must estimate reliability using empirical data. One estimate of reliability is the correlation coefficient for the relationship between two parallel tests. This type of reliability is also called equivalence. We begin this chapter with a discussion of the procedures for conducting a reliability assessment based on parallel tests. We then discuss procedures for evaluating other types of reliability, and we end the chapter with a presentation of generalizability theory.

Methods of Reliability Assessment

Equivalence

One estimate of reliability is the correlation between parallel tests. This type of reliability is referred to as equivalence or alternative-forms reliability. As its name implies, the reliability coefficient is estimated using parallel or alternative forms of the same instrument to assess the degree to which they are equivalent. If a researcher wanted to use the parallel-tests method to estimate the reliability of a scale to measure the degree to which mothers are involved in the daily lives of their children (maternal involvement), he or she could develop two forms of the instrument, each containing maternal involvement items. The best approach for developing the two forms is to write a sufficient number of items and then randomly select items for each form. Because the items would be selected from the same set, the researcher could assume that the two forms of the instrument have the same characteristics, and the random selection of items for each form would help ensure equivalence.

To gather data for a test of equivalence, the researcher administers both forms to the same group of respondents. The respondents complete one form followed immediately, or within a relatively short time period, by the second. Using the scores on the two forms, a correlation coefficient is computed and used as the estimate of reliability.

Equation 10.1

$$r_{x1x2} = r_{ot}^2 .$$

where

r_{x1x2} = the correlation between the two forms, and
r_{ot}^2 = the reliability coefficient.

The SPSS procedures for computing the correlation coefficient were presented in Chapter Eight. Table 10.1 presents the SPSS printout for the correlation coefficient between two forms of a scale that measures maternal involvement. Both forms are completed by adolescents, who evaluate the extent to which their mothers are involved in their daily lives.

The reliability coefficient, also called the coefficient of equivalence, is equal in value to the correlation coefficient, although its values range from 0 to 1 instead of from -1 to $+1$. Lower values of the reliability coefficient are associated with greater amounts

TABLE 10.1. SPSS PRINTOUT SHOWING THE RESULTS OF PARALLEL TEST RELIABILITY ASSESSMENT.

Correlations

		Form 1	Form 2
Form 1	Pearson Correlation	1	
	Sig. (2-tailed)	.	
	N	559	
Form 2	Pearson Correlation	.756[a]	1
	Sig. (2-tailed)	.000	.
	N	553	557

[a] Correlation is significant at the 0.01 level.

of random error, and higher values with less random error. In the present example, the reliability coefficient of .756 indicates that about 76 percent of the variance in the scale is due to true-score variance and 24 percent is due to error-score variance.

The parallel-tests approach to estimating reliability is most intuitive, because it follows directly from CTT. Despite its appeal, there are several issues that make the use of this approach impractical for behavioral scientists. Perhaps the most important issue is the difficulty of constructing a large number of items from which to randomly select those necessary to form two versions of a scale. Developing two forms of a test is relatively easy when one is assessing mathematical concepts such as the addition of two numbers. In such a case, the developer has many choices for the items. The task is much more difficult when one is developing measures of health-related variables. Behavioral scientists generally strive to develop a core set of items that adequately assesses a variable and include these items in one instrument. In addition, the researcher must consider the time and expense of collecting data twice from the same participants. If the instruments are not administered on the same day, the researcher must make arrangements for the second administration. Locating participants and providing incentives to complete the second instrument consumes staff time and costs money.

Stability

A second approach to estimating reliability is to assess the stability of the scores over time. A reliable instrument is one whose items respondents answer the same way every time they complete it. The method used to assess stability is referred to as the test-retest method. In this approach, respondents complete the same instrument twice, and a correlation coefficient is computed for the relationship between the scores on the instrument completed the first time and those from the second administration. Using CTT, it is assumed that if no random errors are present, the correlation between the two tests will be perfect. However, random error reduces the strength of the correlation. As with parallel tests, the correlation coefficient between the two administrations of the same instrument can be used as an estimate of reliability.

Equation 10.2

$$r_{x1x2} = r_{ot}^2.$$

where

r_{x1x2} = the correlation between the scores of the instrument obtained at two different times, and

r_{ot}^2 = the reliability coefficient.

The interpretation of the reliability coefficient for stability is similar to that for parallel tests. If the scores are consistent and the observed score is a reflection of the true score, there should be a high degree of correlation between the scores on the two administrations. The extent to which the coefficient is less than perfect provides an indication of the amount of error present. As with parallel tests, the reliability coefficient ranges from 0 to 1; lower values are associated with greater amounts of random error and higher values with less random error. The test-retest reliability coefficient is sometimes referred to as the coefficient of stability. Table 10.2 presents the results of test-retest for the maternal involvement scale, which was completed by adolescents twice, three months apart. The correlation is .518, indicating roughly equal amounts of true- and error-score variance.

TABLE 10.2. SPSS PRINTOUT SHOWING THE RESULTS OF TEST-RETEST RELIABILITY ASSESSMENT.

		Time 1	Time 2
Time 1	Pearson Correlation Sig. (2-tailed) N	1 . 560	
Time 2	Pearson Correlation Sig. (2-tailed) N	.518[a] .000 552	1 . 558

[a] Correlation is significant at the 0.01 level.

As with the parallel-tests approach, a major disadvantage of the test-retest relia-bility method is the need to administer the instrument a second time. The expense and time commitments for both staff and participants make the method unappealing. When test-retest reliability is conducted within the context of instrument testing, it is usually done with a subsample of the larger sample for the study. Underestimation of reliability may occur for a few reasons. If there is a long period of time between the two administrations of the instrument, changes may have occurred in the variable being measured. These changes inflate the differences between scores, reducing the consistency of scores over time. This is likely the reason for the low test-retest relia-bility of the maternal involvement scale. The three-month time period between ad-ministrations is rather long. It is possible that over this period of time, some mothers became more involved with their adolescents and others less involved. These changes would be reflected in the adolescents' responses to the items, some obtaining higher scores on the scale than the first time and others obtaining lower scores. These changes in scores result in a lower reliability coefficient. Likewise, if a researcher wanted to as-sess the stability of a knowledge test for hypertension and administered the test twice, six months apart, it is possible that some respondents would become more informed about hypertension during the time between administrations. These individuals would obtain higher scores on the second administration, and the changes in their scores would result in a lower reliability coefficient. It is also possible for the respondents to change their behavior as a result of answering questions on an instrument the first time. This change, referred to as reactivity, is reflected in their scores the second time the instrument is administered. For example, parents who answer items related to talk-ing to their children about sex might realize that they should be talking more about such topics with their children. On the second administration of the scale, their an-swers would reflect a change in behavior precipitated by the completion of the in-strument the first time. Lower reliability coefficients are sometimes misinterpreted as measurement instability when in fact they are due to changes in the amount of the variable.

The test-retest method could overestimate reliability as well. Recall that people are likely to answer ambiguous items differently if they are asked to respond to such items a second time. One would expect that the consistency of responses for such items would be low over time and would be reflected in the reliability coefficient. However, if the time between administrations of an instrument is too short, respondents tend to remember how they answered items the first time they completed the instrument and to answer in the same manner the second time. Reliability coefficients for these items are likely to be inflated. Likewise, there is a tendency among participants to approach testing in a similar manner on different occasions, and this tendency can inflate the re-liability coefficient. In this regard, the parallel-tests method is superior because there are few memory effects that can inflate reliability estimates.

When using test-retest, the researcher must consider the stability of the variable being measured. Some human conditions, such as motivation, anxiety, depression, and happiness, are situation-specific. A student who is anxious before a major exam will likely score high on an anxiety measure before the exam and lower after the exam. Some variables change more slowly. Exercise self-efficacy may improve over time when a person feels successful in maintaining a walking program. Other variables, such as IQ, are more enduring. When one is considering the test-retest measure, the rate of change of the variable must be considered in determining the length of time between administrations of the instruments. Most authors suggest a minimum of two weeks to reduce the effects of memory and no more than one month to reduce the chance of change in the amount of the phenomenon reported (Nunnally & Bernstein, 1994). Test-retest is generally not recommended for variables that show change over short periods (for example, test anxiety, which is a transient state).

The time between administrations of the instrument and the stability of the variable affect the reliability coefficient and must be taken into consideration when one is interpreting reliability. For stability, a reliability coefficient of .70 is generally considered acceptable, .80 is better, and .90 or higher is excellent (Nunnally & Bernstein, 1994). Although we focus on scales in this text, test-retest is a useful approach for assessing stability of responses to single-item questions found on surveys.

Internal Consistency

The difficulties inherent in the parallel-tests and test-retest approaches to estimating reliability have led to the development of methods to estimate reliability from a single administration of an instrument. In these approaches, the objective is to estimate reliability from the assessment of correlations among items within the test or scale, or internal consistency. Instead of using the correlation of items between two forms or two administrations of an instrument as an estimate of reliability, this approach uses the correlations among items within an instrument to estimate reliability. Thus, a necessary criterion for computing an internal-consistency reliability coefficient is that the measure must consist of more than one item that measures the variable. The most common forms of internal consistency are split-half, coefficient alpha, and Kuder-Richardson-20 (Kuder & Richardson, 1937).

Split-Half. In the split-half method, a reliability estimate is obtained by correlating the scores of items from two equal parts of a single instrument. Conceptually, this method is similar to the parallel-tests approach in that each half of the instrument is considered to be one form of a test. To gather data for the assessment of split-half reliability, the researcher administers an instrument once to a group of respondents. The items are then divided into two halves using one of several methods:

- Odd-numbered and even-numbered items
- The first half and second half of the list of items
- Items randomly selected for each half

A correlation coefficient is computed and provides an estimate of reliability for an instrument half as long as the original. Splitting a test in half results in a test that is half as long as the original, and because shorter tests generally have lower internal-consistency reliability than longer ones, an adjustment is needed to reflect the reliability of the total instrument.

The Spearman-Brown formula (Brown, 1910; Spearman, 1910) is used for this adjustment and is presented in Equation 10.3.

Equation 10.3

$$Tr_{ot}^2 = \frac{2Hr_{ot}^2}{1 + Hr_{ot}^2}$$

where

Tr_{ot}^2 = the reliability for the total test, and
Hr_{ot}^2 = the reliability for one half of the test.

Expressed in words, the total reliability is equal to twice the reliability for half the instrument divided by the sum of 1 plus the reliability for half the instrument.

Suppose that our maternal involvement scale is composed of six items. We randomly divide the items into two equal groups of three items each. We first calculate a Pearson correlation coefficient using the two parts of the scale and obtain a correlation coefficient of .587. We then make the following adjustment:

$$Tr_{ot}^2 = \frac{2(.587)}{1 + .587} = \frac{1.17}{1.59} = .74$$

The reliability for the scale composed of six items is .74. Note that the reliability coefficient of .74 is greater than .587, the correlation between the two halves. Exhibit 10.1 presents the results of a split-half reliability that was computed using SPSS for the maternal involvement scale. SPSS uses more than one equation for the computation of split-half; these are shown in the exhibit. Notice the correlation between the two halves (1) and the reliability coefficient for the total test (2).

The commands at the top of page 183 will calculate a split-half reliability.

The reliability coefficient for the split-half test is interpreted in the same way as the parallel-tests and test-retest reliability coefficients. Split-half values range from 0 to 1; values near 0 indicate very low reliability and values near 1 indicate very high reliability.

To compute a split-half reliability:

From the Data Editor Screen:

√Analyze. . . .Scale. . . .√Reliability Analysis

    Highlight and transfer scale items from L→R column

    Select Split-half from the pull down menu

    √OK

EXHIBIT 10.1. SPSS PRINTOUT SHOWING THE RESULTS OF A SPLIT-HALF RELIABILITY ASSESSMENT FOR THE MATERNAL INVOLVEMENT SCALE.

Case Processing Summary

		N	%
Cases	Valid	560	98.9
	Excluded [a]	6	1.1
	Total	566	100.0

Reliability Statistics

Cronbach's Alpha	Part 1	Value	.697
		N of items	3[b]
	Part 2	Value	.582
		N of items	3[c]
	Total N of items		6
Correlation Between Forms			.587
Spearman-Brown	Equal Length		.740
Coefficient	Unequal Length		.740
Guttman Split-Half Coefficient			.739

1. Correlation between halves

2. Reliability coefficient

[a] Listwise deletion based on all variables in the procedure.

[b] The items are "Count on Mother to help with problems," "Mother helps you with your school work," "Mother spends time talking to you."

[c] The items are "Mother spends time getting to know your friends," "Mother does fun things with you," "Mother knows where you are after school."

The advantage of the split-half reliability test is that it requires only one administration of the instrument. The disadvantage is that there are many different ways in which a set of items can be divided into two equal parts. For example, there are twenty possible ways for a six-item scale to be divided into two equal parts. The reliability estimates for these twenty divisions are likely to vary, and in some cases these differences could be large. Therefore, the reliability estimate depends heavily on the items that make up the two halves. Largely because of this deficiency in computing the reliability estimate, behavioral scientists rarely use the split-half method today. We mention it here because of its conceptual similarity to parallel tests and because it was widely used before computer packages became available.

Coefficient Alpha. A second approach to measuring internal-consistency reliability is the calculation of coefficient alpha (Cronbach, 1951). In this approach, each item is correlated with every other item on the instrument. Coefficient alpha is computed by taking the average of the individual item-to-item correlations and adjusting for the number of items. The advantage of this approach as compared to split-half is that only one value of coefficient alpha can be computed for an instrument. Coefficient alpha can be computed using either the correlation or the variance-covariance matrix. The two equations for computing coefficient alpha are presented following with examples.

The first equation uses the mean of the correlation coefficients among the items (item-item correlations) in the computation of coefficient alpha.

Equation 10.4

$$\alpha = \frac{Np}{\left[1 + p\,(N-1)\right]}$$

where

α = alpha coefficient,
N = number of items, and
p = mean interitem correlation.

As an example, Table 10.3 presents a correlation matrix for six items on a scale that measures maternal involvement.

The first step in the computation of alpha is to calculate the mean interitem correlation. To do this, the correlations among the items, as shown in an item-item correlation matrix, are summed and then divided by the total number of correlations. (Remember that each interitem correlation is presented twice in a full matrix. For this equation, only one of each interitem correlation is included; that is, only the values

TABLE 10.3. CORRELATION MATRIX FOR THE MATERNAL INVOLVEMENT SCALE.

	MOM1	MOM2	MOM3	MOM4	MOM5	MOM6
MOM1	1.0000					
MOM2	.4984	1.0000				
MOM3	.4301	.3806	1.0000			
MOM4	.2863	.2558	.4175	1.0000		
MOM5	.4174	.4070	.4868	.3947	1.0000	
MOM6	.3100	.3053	.2834	.2514	.3578	1.0000

below [or above] the diagonal). In this example, the fifteen interitem correlations are summed as follows:

$$(.4984 + .4301 + \ldots \ldots + .2514 + .3578 = 5.481),$$

and the sum is divided by 15 (the number of item-item correlations) to obtain the mean interitem correlation

$$\frac{5.481}{15} = .3655.$$

The mean interitem correlation is .3655. We then substitute .366 in Equation 10.4 to compute alpha:

$$\alpha = \frac{6(.366)}{1 + .366(6 - 1)} = \frac{2.20}{2.83} = .78.$$

(It is important to remember the fundamental rules of algebra when you are using this equation. The element $p(N - 1)$ must be computed before adding 1.)

Two primary elements of Equation 10.4 are the number of items (N) and the mean interitem correlation (p). If the value of either one changes without a change in the other, alpha will change accordingly. For example, if we increase the number of items on our maternal involvement scale from six to ten while the mean interitem correlation remains .366, coefficient alpha increases, as shown here:

$$\alpha = \frac{10(.366)}{1 + .366(10 - 1)} = \frac{3.66}{4.29} = .85.$$

TABLE 10.4. VARIANCE-COVARIANCE MATRIX.

	Item 1	Item 2	Item 3	Item 4
Item 1	**VAR**	CoVar	CoVar	CoVar
Item 2	CoVar	**VAR**	CoVar	CoVar
Item 3	CoVar	CoVar	**VAR**	CoVar
Item 4	CoVar	CoVar	CoVar	**VAR**

Likewise, if the mean interitem correlation increases from .366 to .60, alpha also increases:

$$\alpha = \frac{6\,(.60)}{1 + .60\,(6-1)} = \frac{3.6}{4.0} = .90.$$

Cronbach's Alpha. The second equation for calculating a coefficient alpha is based on the variance-covariance matrix (Cronbach, 1951). To create the matrix for a set of items, a variance is calculated for each item and a covariance for each item with every other item on the test. These variances and covariances can be shown in a matrix, called a variance-covariance matrix or simply a covariance matrix (Table 10.4). Variances are represented in the diagonal and covariances are in off-diagonal locations.

Using the variances and covariances, alpha is computed as follows.

Equation 10.5

$$\alpha = \frac{N}{N-1}\left[1 - \frac{\sum \sigma_i^2}{\sum \sigma_i^2 + 2\left(\sum \sigma_{ij}^2\right)}\right],$$

where

α = alpha coefficient,
N = number of items,
$\sum \sigma_i^2$ = sum of item variances, and
$2\left(\sum \sigma_{ij}^2\right)$ = twice the sum of the covariances below (or above) the diagonal.

Another way to show the equation is

$$\alpha = \left(\frac{n}{n-1}\right)\left(1 - \frac{sum\ of\ diagonals\ of\ elements}{sum\ of\ all\ elements}\right).$$

The equation states that the sum of the variances (these are on the diagonal) is divided by the sum of the variances plus twice the sum of the covariance for each

TABLE 10.5. VARIANCE-COVARIANCE FOR THE MATERNAL INVOLVEMENT SCALE.

	MOM1	MOM2	MOM3	MOM4	MOM5	MOM6
MOM1	.6252					
MOM2	.3496	.7870				
MOM3	.2801	.2781	.6784			
MOM4	.2678	.2684	.4067	1.3989		
MOM5	.2758	.3018	.3351	.3902	.6984	
MOM6	.1995	.2204	.1900	.2420	.2434	.6623

item-item pair (same as summing all numbers in the matrix). This result is subtracted from 1 and then adjusted for the number of items on the test $[N/(N-1)]$.

Table 10.5 presents the variances and covariances for the six items on the maternal involvement scale. The sum of the variances is found by adding the numbers on the diagonal.

$$.6252 + .7870 + .6784 + 1.3984 + .6984 + .6623 = 4.85$$

The sum of the covariances is found by adding all the numbers below the diagonal as follows.

$$.3496 + .2801 + ... .2420 + .2434 = 4.25$$

These values are entered into the Equation 10.5 as follows.

$$\alpha = \frac{6}{6-1}\left[1 - \frac{4.85}{4.85 + 2(4.25)}\right] = (1.20)(1 - .363) = (1.20)(.637) = .76.$$

The values of coefficient alpha (.78 and .76) derived from Equations 10.4 and 10.5 are similar, because the correlation matrix is derived from the covariance matrix (correlations are standardized covariance scores). The values will be very similar when the items have similar variances; discrepancies in the values occur when the item variances are dissimilar. Because Equation 10.4 uses standardized scores (correlation coefficients), the alpha calculated from it is referred to as the standardized alpha. Equation 10.5 uses raw scores in the calculation of alpha and is referred to as the unstandardized alpha. The unstandardized alpha is sometimes referred to as Cronbach's alpha, in honor of Lee Cronbach (1951), who first proposed this internal-consistency approach to reliability. Exhibit 10.2 presents the SPSS printout for the alpha coefficient for the maternal involvement scale.

The following commands are used to compute a coefficient alpha.

To compute an alpha coefficient:

From the Data Editor Screen:

√Analyze. . . .Scale. . . .√Reliability analysis

    Highlight and transfer scale items L→R column

    Alpha is the default in the drop down box

    √OK

EXHIBIT 10.2. SPSS PRINTOUT FOR THE ALPHA COEFFICIENT FOR THE MATERNAL INVOLVEMENT SCALE.

Case Processing Summary

		N	%
Cases	Valid	560	98.9
	Excluded[a]	6	1.1
	Total	566	100.0

Reliability Statistics

Cronbach's Alpha	N of Items
.764	6

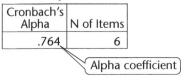

Alpha coefficient

[a] Listwise deletion based on all variables in the procedure.

The range of values for coefficient alpha is the same as for the other forms of reliability we have discussed: values range between 0 and 1, and values closer to 1 reflect higher levels of interrelatedness among the items. The more interrelated the items are, the greater the reliability. Standardized alpha is used when item standard scores are summed to form scale scores. The unstandardized alpha (covariance matrix) is used when raw scores of items are summed to form scales and takes into account differences in the item standard deviations. The value of unstandardized alpha is generally slightly lower than that of standardized alpha.

The internal consistency of a scale is sometimes confused with the homogeneity of a scale (Green, Lissitz, & Mulaik, 1977). The term *internal consistency* refers to the interrelatedness of items. The term *homogeneity* refers to the unidimensionality of a scale. A scale is said to be unidimensional when all its items measure the same variable. By definition, unidimensional scales will demonstrate high interrelatedness among items. However, the reverse is not always true. Items can demonstrate a high interrelatedness as evidenced by a high alpha coefficient, yet measure more than one dimension. Scales that measure two or more dimensions are called multidimensional scales. Though a coefficient alpha will provide an indication of the interrelatedness of items, an alpha does not provide an index of dimensionality.

Kuder-Richardson Formula 20. The third equation used to assess internal consistency reliability is Kuder-Richardson Formula 20 (KR20) (Kuder & Richardson, 1937). This equation is named after the two men who developed it. KR20 differs from coefficient alpha in that it is used to assess interrelatedness among dichotomous items— items that provide only two possible response options, such as *yes/no*, *agree/disagree*, or *true/false*.

The procedure for collecting data is the same as that for split-half and coefficient alpha estimation. The scale is administered once to a group of participants. The following formula, which is based on the proportion of responses in each category, is used to compute KR20:

Equation 10.6

$$KR20 = \frac{N}{N-1}\left(1 - \frac{\sum pq}{\sigma_t^2}\right),$$

where

$KR20$ = The Kuder Richardson 20 coefficient
Σ = sum
N = number of dichotomous items,
p = proportion of correct (or positive) responses,
$q = 1 - p$ = proportion of incorrect (or negative) responses, and
σ_t^2 = variance of the total test.

Suppose that a researcher administers an HIV knowledge test to a group of college students. Each of the five items requires an answer of *true* or *false*. Each correct item is coded 1; each incorrect item, 0. To calculate a KR20 using the above formula, the researcher first must calculate, for each item, the proportion of respondents who answered it correctly (p) and the proportion that answered it incorrectly (q equal to $1 - p$). The two proportions are multiplied for each item and then summed across all items ($\sum pq$). This number is divided by the variance of the total test. The resulting number is subtracted from 1, and the result is multiplied by $N/N - 1$.

For the five-item HIV knowledge test, the $\sum pq$ is .872 and the variance is 1.69. The value of KR20 for this test is .643 as computed below.

$$KR20 = \frac{5}{5-1}\left(1 - \frac{.872}{1.69}\right) = (1.25)(.515) = .643.$$

Possible values of KR20 range from 0 to 1; those closer to 1 indicate higher levels of reliability. Exhibit 10.3 presents the SPSS printout for an HIV knowledge test for college students. The SPSS output will look the same as that for coefficient alpha and the term *alpha* will be used because the KR20 formula is equivalent to Equation 10.5.

The following SPSS commands are used to calculate a KR20 coefficient.

To compute a KR20:

From the Data Editor Screen:

√Analyze. . . .Scale. . . .√Reliability analysis

    Highlight and transfer scale items L→R column.

    Alpha is the default and is used for KR20

    √OK

EXHIBIT 10.3. SPSS PRINTOUT OF THE RESULTS OF A KR20 FOR AN HIV KNOWLEDGE TEST.

Case Processing Summary

		N	%
Cases	Valid	221	100.0
	Excluded[a]	0	.0
	Total	220	100.0

Reliability Statistics

Cronbach's Alpha	N of Items
.643	5

Kuder-Richardson 20

Note: When KR20 is used to assess the reliability of a knowledge test, as it was used here with the HIV Knowledge Test, the reliability of the test can be underestimated if the test items are of different levels of difficulty. Likewise, a shorter test will have a lower reliability coefficient than a longer test with items of similar difficulty.

[a]Listwise deletion based on all variables in the procedure.

Factors Associated with Coefficient Alpha

Test Length and Interitem Correlation

We have said previously that the number of items on an instrument affect the value of internal-consistency coefficients. Table 10.6 shows a good example of what happens when the interitem correlation increases (rows) and the number of items increases (columns). The lowest reliabilities, in the upper left part of the table, are for scales with a small number of items and a low interitem correlation. Higher values of alpha, associated with scales that have more items and higher interitem correlations, are in the lower right.

Test Adjustments to Increase Alpha

If the reliability of a scale is lower than desired, a researcher can use the following equation, a variant of the Spearman-Brown formula, to determine the reliability when items are added. Using this approach, the researcher asks what the reliability of a test twice or three or more times as long will be. N in this equation refers to multiples of length (two or three times as long) and not number of items.

Equation 10.7

$$Lr_{ot}^2 = \frac{Nr_{ot}^2}{1 + (N-1)\,r_{ot}^2},$$

where

$Lr_{ot}^2 =$ the reliability of the longer test,
$r_{ot}^2 =$ the reliability of the original scale, and
$N =$ number of multiples of the original length of the instrument.

TABLE 10.6. VALUES OF CRONBACH'S ALPHA FOR VARIOUS COMBINATIONS OF DIFFERENT NUMBER OF ITEMS AND DIFFERENT AVERAGE INTERITEM CORRELATIONS.

Number of Items	Average Interitem Correlation					
	0	.2	.4	.6	.8	1.0
2	.000	.333	.572	.750	.889	1.000
4	.000	.500	.727	.857	.941	1.000
6	.000	.600	.800	.900	.960	1.000
8	.000	.666	.842	.924	.970	1.000
10	.000	.714	.870	.938	.976	1.000

Source: Carmines & Zeller, 1979, p. 46. Reprinted by permission of Sage Publications Inc.

Suppose a researcher has developed a four-item scale to measure health-related quality of life. The alpha coefficient for these four items is .40. The researcher believes that he or she can add twelve items; this increases the length five times (from four to twenty items).

$$\frac{5(.40)}{\left[1 + (5 - 1).40\right]} = \frac{2}{1 + 1.6} = .77.$$

The reliability of the original scale is .40. By adding twelve items, the researcher can increase the reliability to .77. The trick with this equation is to remember that computation is based on multiples of the original number of items and not on the number of items itself. Thus, you can calculate the expected reliability for a test twice as long or three times as long, and so on.

The next equation can be used to tell the researcher how many additional items are needed to obtain a desired level of reliability. However, as in the preceding equation, N is equal to the number by which the length of a test must be multiplied to reach the desired level of reliability.

Equation 10.8

$$N = \frac{Lr_{ot}^2\left(1 - r_{ot}^2\right)}{r_{ot}^2\left(1 - Lr_{ot}^2\right)}$$

where

N = the number by which the length of the test must be multiplied to give the desired reliability,
r_{ot}^2 = the existing reliability, and
Lr_{ot}^2 = the desired reliability.

Another way of writing the equation is:

$$N = \frac{(desired\ reliability)(1 - existing\ reliability)}{(existing\ reliability)(1 - desired\ reliability)}.$$

Suppose that the researcher would like his or her new four-item measure of health-related quality of life to have a reliability coefficient of .80. Using Equation 10.8, the researcher can calculate how long the scale must be.

$$N = \frac{.80(1 - .40)}{.40(1 - .80)} = \frac{.48}{.08} = 6.$$

To achieve a reliability of .80, the researcher must increase the length of the test by a factor of 6 to create a twenty-four-item scale. An assumption of this equation and the previous equation is that the items added are comparable in quality to the original items. Adding weak items that do not adequately measure the construct will improve the reliability somewhat but not to the extent desired.

Standards of Reliability

Nunnally and Bernstein (1994) and others suggest that an alpha coefficient of .70 or greater be used as a standard to estimate reliability. A coefficient of less than .70 is considered to be low reliability; one higher than .70 is considered at least adequate. However, it is important to note that .70 should not be the only standard used to assess reliability. The number of items and the mean interitem correlation should be considered as well. A reliability coefficient of .80 reflects a higher interrelatedness among items than a coefficient of .60 only when the numbers of items on the scales are equivalent. However, when the scale with a coefficient of .60 has few items and the scale with a reliability of .80 has a large number of items, the mean interitem correlation among items on the shorter scale could be greater than that on the longer scale. If this is the case, the shorter scale, with the lower alpha value, actually demonstrates higher interrelatedness among items. (See Table 10.6)

Alpha assesses the degree to which there is interrelatedness among the items, but does not give any information about the stability of the test over time. Some measures will demonstrate high internal consistency and low stability and vice versa. Thus, most psychometricians suggest estimating stability as well as internal consistency.

Item Analysis

The SPSS commands for computing a coefficient alpha, presented earlier in this chapter, give only the value of the alpha. The reliability analysis of SPSS can be used to generate information about the characteristics of the items and their association with one another. This information can be used to make decisions about retaining or deleting individual items. The process of reviewing the characteristics of items and their association with each other and the scale is referred to as item analysis. In this section, we refer to Exhibit 10.4, which is the printout for an item analysis of the six items presented earlier on the maternal involvement scale. The SPSS commands for generating this printout are as shown in the following box.

To obtain item statisitics:

From the Data Editor Screen:

√Analyze. . . .Scale. . . .√Reliability analysis

    Highlight and transfer variables from L→R column.

    √Statistics (dialog box)

        √Descriptives (Item, Scale, Scale if item deleted)

        √Summaries (Means, Variances, Covariances, Correlations)

        √Inter-item (Correlations, Covariances)

        √Continue

    √OK

In Exhibit 10.4, the first section gives us the number of cases processed. Reliability will be computed only for cases in which all the items on the scale have been answered. Thus, the number of cases may be smaller than the total sample size. The second section gives the values of both the coefficient alpha computed with the covariance matrix and the standardized item alpha computed from the correlation matrix. The value of the unstandardized coefficient, .764 (generally rounded to two decimal places, .76), is considered reasonable for a six-item scale.

The section labeled Item Statistics gives the name of each item along with its mean, its standard deviation, and the sample size. The researcher can review the means and standard deviations and determine whether or not they are reasonable. If the means are greater or less than the expected high and low values of the response scale or seem odd, data entry errors may have occurred or the negatively worded items may not have been recoded during analysis. In the present case, a five-point scale was used, and the means of all the items are less than 5, as expected. However, the means of five items are greater than 4, indicating that respondents had a tendency to choose responses at the high end of the scale. The standard deviations indicate some variability around the mean, but not much. A concern with these items is that there appears to be a ceiling effect. That is, most adolescents are selecting responses at the high end of the scale. The opposite of the ceiling effect is the floor effect, in which most participants choose responses at the low end of the scale. To improve these items, researchers can rewrite the items to make them more difficult for participants to give either strong positive or strong negative responses.

EXHIBIT 10.4. SPSS PRINTOUT FOR USE IN ITEM ANALYSIS FOR THE MATERNAL INVOLVEMENT SCALE.

Case Processing Summary

		N	%
Cases	Valid	560	98.9
	Excluded [a]	6	1.1
	Total	566	100.0

[a] Listwise deletion based on all variables in the procedure.

Coefficient based on standardized items (item responses converted to z scores).

Reliability Statistics

Cronbach's Alpha	Cronbach's Alpha Based on Standardized Items	N of Items
.764	.776	6

Alpha based on convariance formula; Cronbach's alpha

Descriptive statistics and sample size; only complete cases included

Item Statistics

	Mean	Std. Deviation	N
1. Count on mother to help with problems	4.4696	.79069	560
2. Mother helps you with your school work	4.2607	.88713	560
3. Mother spends time talking to you	4.2982	.82362	560
4. Mother spends time getting to know your friends	3.7464	1.18276	560
5. Mother does fun things with you	4.3036	.83569	560
6. Mother knows where you are after school	4.3821	.81381	560

EXHIBIT 10.4. *(continued)*

Interitem correlations;
inspect for low and
high values

Interitem Correlation Matrix

	Count on mother to help with problems	Mother helps you with your school work	Mother spends time talking to you	Mother spends time getting to know your friends	Mother does fun things with you	Mother knows where you are after school
1. Count on mother to help with problems	1.000	.498	.430	.286	.417	.310
2. Mother helps you with your school work	.498	1.000	.381	.256	.407	.305
3. Mother spends time talking to you	.430	.381	1.000	.417	.487	.283
4. Mother spends time getting to know your friends	.286	.256	.417	1.000	.395	.251
5. Mother does fun things with you	.417	.407	.487	.395	1.000	.358
6. Mother knows where you are after school	.310	.305	.283	.251	.358	1.000

The covariance matrix is calculated and used in the analysis.

Matrix used to
calculate Cronbach's
alpha

Interitem Covariance Matrix

	Count on mother to help with problems	Mother helps you with your school work	Mother spends time talking to you	Mother spends time getting to know your friends	Mother does fun things with you	Mother knows where you are after school
1. Count on mother to help with problems	.625	.350	.280	.268	.276	.199
2. Mother helps you with your school work	.350	.787	.278	.268	.302	.220
3. Mother spends time talking to you	.280	.278	.678	.407	.335	.190
4. Mother spends time getting to know your friends	.268	.268	.407	1.399	.390	.242
5. Mother does fun things with you	.276	.302	.335	.390	.698	.243
6. Mother knows where you are after school	.199	.220	.190	.242	.243	.662

The covariance matrix is calculated and used in the analysis.

EXHIBIT 10.4. *(continued)*

Scale and item-descriptive statistics; note mean interitem correlation

Summary Item Statistics

	Mean	Minimum	Maximum	Range	Maximum/ Minimum	Variance	N of items
Item Means	4.234	3.746	4.470	.723	1.193	.065	6
Item Variances	.808	.625	1.399	.774	2.238	.087	6
Interitem Covariances	.283	.190	.407	.217	2.141	.004	6
Interitem Correlations	.366	.251	.498	.247	1.983	.006	6

The covariance matrix is calculated and used in the analysis.

This value can be used to compute alpha using the correlation formula

Correlation of item with total scores; inspect to identify correlations below .20

Item-Total Statistics

	Scale Mean If Item Deleted	Scale Variance If Item Deleted	Corrected Item-Total Correlation	Squared Multiple Correlation	Cronbach's Alpha If Item Deleted
1. Count on mother to help with problems	20.9911	9.977	.550	.346	.721
2. Mother helps you with your school work	21.2000	9.724	.513	.318	.728
3. Mother spends time talking to you	21.1625	9.689	.581	.355	.712
4. Mother spends time getting to know your friends	21.1743	8.798	.449	.232	.760
5. Mother does fun things with you	21.1571	9.557	.598	.365	.707
6. Mother knows where you are after school	21.0786	10.495	.415	.182	.751

R^2 when item is dependent variable and others independent variables

New alpha value if item is deleted; values increase for poor items.

EXHIBIT 10.4. *(continued)*

Scale Statistics

Mean	Variance	Std. Deviation	N of Items
25.4607	13.347	3.65339	6

   The next two sections present the correlation and covariance matrices. The variance-covariance matrix provides information about the covariance between items. The values in the matrix are used to compute the coefficient alpha. Although this matrix provides the same information as the correlation matrix, it is difficult to interpret because it is not standardized. The correlation matrix provides the relationships in standardized form and makes it easier to discern the stronger and weaker relationships. The correlation matrix provides information about the interrelatedness of items. Items that are closely associated will have high values and those with weak relationships will have low values. Generally, in scale development, values between .20 and .80 are considered ideal (Nunnally & Bernstein, 1994). Correlations of less than .20 generally indicate an item that has little in common with other items, whereas correlations above .80 indicate redundancy. During the initial review, the developer identifies these items for a more thorough review, to be conducted after other tests are performed.

   In the present example, the correlations range from .256 to .498, so they are all within the suggested range. Thus, none of the items would be identified as problem items at this stage of the analysis.

   An overview of the scale statistics is presented in the Summary Item Statistics section. A review of this section yields information to determine whether the values are within the expected range. Perhaps the most important number in this section is the mean interitem correlation. This provides some indication of the interrelatedness among items; a higher value indicates greater interrelatedness. In the present example, the interitem mean correlation is .366.

   The next section provides statistics on the association of each item with the total scale. This information is used to assess how each individual item is functioning within the context of the scale. The first column lists the items, the second column gives the new mean value of the scale if the corresponding item is deleted, and the third column gives the new variance. The fourth column is the column of most interest in scale development. This column provides an indication of how closely each item is associated with the total scale. For this calculation, the total scale is composed of all the remaining items and does not include the item under consideration. If an item is strongly associated with the total scale, the value of the correlation will be higher than if it is not associated or has a weak association. Items that show a weak correlation (<.20) are identified for more thorough review (Nunnally & Bernstein, 1994). Likewise, items that show a very high correlation (>.80) are identified for more thorough review. The information from this column is used in conjunction with the information in the last column to decide the fate of each item. The last column gives the new alpha value if the item is deleted. If the alpha is higher than the current alpha given at the top of the printout, the item is considered weak and is marked for further review. If the new alpha is lower than the current alpha, the item is retained, because to delete it would reduce the value of alpha.

The next-to-last column (Squared Multiple Correlation) provides information on how the item is related to the other items in the set. In this calculation, the item functions as the dependent variable and the other items as independent variables. The value indicates the amount of variance explained in the item by all the remaining items. Higher values indicate greater association.

In the present example, the corrected item-total correlations range from .415 to .598 and the value of alpha decreases when any of the items is deleted from the scale. Thus, none of the items would be considered for removal.

The final section includes a summary of the scale statistics—mean, variance, standard deviation, and number of items

A review of the maternal involvement scale items shows that the all the interitem correlations are within the acceptable range as are the item-total correlations, and the mean interitem correlation is moderate. Moreover, none of the values for alpha increase when an item is deleted. Based on this information, the researcher would not eliminate any of the items. If, however, one or more items did not meet the criteria, the researcher could (1) eliminate the item from the scale, (2) rephrase the item to make it more consistent with the other items, or (3) keep the item in the scale for further evaluation. If the item(s) continues to perform poorly, the researcher may decide later to eliminate or rephrase it.

Intrarater and Interrater Reliability

So far, we have discussed reliability associated with responses on self-report scales. Scores for some instruments are based on the judgment of observers. In these cases, we use procedures for estimating intrarater and interrater reliability. *Intrarater reliability* refers to agreement, or consistency, among scores assigned by one rater, and *interrater reliability* refers to agreement, or consistency, among scores assigned by two or more raters.

There are a number of research situations in which intrarater or interrater reliability can be used. Situations in which observers view situations and code them according to predetermined rules are very common. These observations might be used to collect data to answer research questions or to evaluate the extent to which project staff are implementing research procedures according to protocol. Consider Megan, a researcher who uses videotape recordings to rate the quality of communication between mothers and daughters. She has trained two observers to view the tapes and to rate the type and quality of the communication. Before the raters begin their task, Megan wants to make certain that they have the same understanding of the task and are rating the tapes in similar ways. To assess interrater reliability, she selects several segments of different tapes showing mother-daughter interaction and asks the observers to rate these segments independently. For each segment, the observers are to record a 1 if the mother-daughter interaction exhibits conflict and a 0 if it does not. The results of their observations for ten tape segments are presented in Table 10.7.

A quick and easy way to determine interrater agreement is to calculate the percentage of agreement by dividing the number of times the raters agreed by the total number of paired observations and multiplying by 100 percent. The total number of paired observations is equal to the number of agreements plus the number of disagreements:

Equation 10.9

$$\text{Percentage of agreement} = \frac{\textit{number of agreements}}{\textit{number of agreements} + \textit{number of disagreements}}.$$

In this example, Observer 1 classified tape segments 5 and 9 as conflict, and Observer 2 did not. Observer 2, however, classified tape segment 8 as conflict, and observer 1 did not. The percentage of agreement for the two raters, as calculated below, is 70 percent.

$$\text{Percentage of agreement} = \frac{7}{7+3} = .7 \times 100 = 70\%.$$

Because this approach does not take chance agreement into consideration, it is generally recommended that the percentage of agreement be at least 90 percent to meet the requirements for interrater agreement. If the level of agreement is less than 90 percent, the researcher should evaluate the reasons behind the ratings and conduct additional training as necessary until the percentage of agreement is 90 percent or more.

Percentage agreement can also be used to assess intrarater agreement. In this case, one observer rates a set of observations on two occasions. The percentage of agreement is computed in the same way: by dividing the number of agreements by the total number of paired observations.

TABLE 10.7. RATINGS OF TWO OBSERVERS ON TEN VIDEOTAPE SEGMENTS.

Tape Segment	Observer 1	Observer 2
1	1	1
2	1	1
3	0	0
4	1	1
5	1	0
6	0	0
7	0	0
8	0	1
9	1	0
10	0	0

Although the percentage-of-agreement approach is easy to calculate and understand, a disadvantage of this approach is that it does not take chance agreement into consideration. A more acceptable statistic is Cohen's K, or kappa (Cohen, 1960), which adjusts the percentage of agreement for agreements based on chance. Table 10.8 presents a cross-tabulation of the data presented in Table 10.7.

The formula for kappa appears in Equation 10.10.

Equation 10.10

$$\kappa = \frac{P_o - P_c}{1 - P_c},$$

where

K = kappa,
P_o = the proportion of the total number of observations in agreement, and
P_c = the proportion of observations in the agreement cells expected by chance given the marginal distributions.

Using the data presented in Table 10.8, P_o is computed by adding the number of observations in the agreement cells (1) and dividing by the total number of observations (2). P_c is computed by first dividing the totals for the row (3) and column (3) for the first condition (conflict) by the overall total number of observations (2) and multiplying them together. This step is followed by dividing the totals for the row (4) and column (3) for the second condition (no conflict) by the total number of observations (2) and multiplying them together. The results of these first two steps are then added together to give the proportion of observations due to chance.

TABLE 10.8. CROSS-TABULATIONS FOR AGREEMENT AMONG OBSERVERS.

	Observer 1		
Observer 2	Conflict	No Conflict	Total
Conflict	$3^{(1)}$	1	$4^{(3)}$
No conflict	2	$4^{(1)}$	$6^{(4)}$
Total	$5^{(3)}$	$5^{(4)}$	$10^{(2)}$

To calculate K, we enter the values for P_o and P_c into Equation 10.10. The calculations for our example are

$$P_o = \frac{3+4}{10} .70,$$

$$P_c = \left(\frac{4}{10}\right)\left(\frac{5}{10}\right) + \left(\frac{6}{10}\right)\left(\frac{5}{10}\right) = \frac{20}{100} + \frac{30}{100} = \frac{50}{100} = .5, \text{ and}$$

$$\kappa = \frac{.7 - .5}{1 - .5} = \frac{.2}{.5} = .4.$$

SPSS commands for computing kappa are shown in the following box.

SPSS output for this data set is displayed in Exhibit 10.5. SPSS also calculates a significance level. In this case, $p = .197$, which means that it is not statistically significant.

The values of K can range from <0 to $+1$, but are typically between 0 and 1. A value of 0 indicates that obtained agreement equals chance agreement and $+1.00$ indicates perfect agreement (Cohen, 1960). Kappa values of .4 to .75 are considered acceptable, and those above .81 are considered strong (Landis & Koch, 1977). As you can see, the kappa value in Table 10.5 (.40) is lower than that for the simple percent

---

To compute Kappa:

From the Data Editor Screen:

√Analyze. . . .Descriptive Statistics. . . .√Crosstabs

    Highlight and transfer one variable from L column→Row(s)

    Highlight and transfer the other variable from L column→Column(s)

    √Statistics (dialogue box)

        √Kappa

        √Continue

  √OK

of agreement computed earlier (.70) and would be considered low interrater reliability. Although a *p* value is computed, the absolute value of kappa (sometimes multiplied by 100 and given as a percentage) is most often used for interpretation.

Intraclass Correlation Coefficient

The intraclass correlation coefficient (ICC) allows the computation of reliability using continuous variables and categorical variables with more than two response choices. Consider our researcher who wants to evaluate the tapes of mother-daughter interactions. To facilitate the coding process, the researcher might hire more than two observers to do the coding. In addition, the researcher might decide that two categories are not sufficient and that the categories should be rated on a five-point scale from *no conflict at all* to *high degree of conflict*. In this case, the ICC can be calculated.

EXHIBIT 10.5. SPSS PRINTOUT WITH THE RESULTS OF KAPPA.

Case Processing Summary

	Cases					
	Valid		Missing		Total	
	N	Percent	N	Percent	N	Percent
obs1* obs2	10	100.0%	0	.0%	10	100.0%

obs1* obs2 Cross-Tabulation

Count

		obs2		
		.00	1.00	Total
obs1	.00	4	1	5
	1.00	2	3	5
Total		6	4	10

Symmetric Measures

	Value	Asymp Std. Error[a]	Approx. T[b]	Approx. Sig.
Measurement of Agreement Kappa N of Valid Cases	.400 10	.284	1.291	.197

[a] Not assuming the null hypothesis.

[b] Using the asymptotic standard error assuming the null hypothesis.

The ICC is defined as the ratio of variance in the variable of interest divided by the total variance, which includes both the variance in the variable plus error variance. There are several forms of the ICC, and consideration of using the ICC depends on the situation and the nature of the variables. We present here the two-way mixed-effect model, the default option in SPSS.

The SPSS commands for computing an intraclass correlation coefficient are shown in the box.

For this analysis, Megan asked three observers to rate each of the ten tapes using a five-point rating scale. The data file for analysis is created so that the raters form the columns and the tape observations form the rows. The ICC of .87 (Exhibit 10.6) indicates a fairly high agreement among the observers in their evaluations of the tape segments. Confidence intervals are generally reported along with the ICC.

To compute ICC:

From the Data Editor Screen:

√Analyze. . . .Scale. . . .√Reliability analysis

    Highlight and transfer variables from L→R column

    √Statistics (dialog box)

        √Intraclass correlation coefficient (Default is two-way mixed and consistency)

        √Continue

√OK

EXHIBIT 10.6. SPSS PRINTOUT OF AN INTRACLASS CORRELATION COEFFICIENT.

Intraclass Correlation Coefficient

	Intraclass Correlation[a]	95% Confidence Interval		F Test with True Value 0			
		Lower Bound	Upper Bound	Value	df1	df2	Sig
Single Measures	.886[b]	.708	.967	24.265	9.0	18	.000
Average Measures	.959[c]	.879	.989	24.265	9.0	18	.000

Note: Two-way mixed effects model where people effects are random and measures effects are fixed.

[a]Type C intraclass correlation coefficients using a consistency definition-the-between-measure variance is excluded from the denominator variance.

[b]The estimator is the same, whether the interaction effect is present or not.

[c]This estimate is computed assuming the interaction effect is absent, because it is not estimable otherwise.

Standard Error of Measurement

In Chapter Nine, we learned that the standard deviation of error scores is referred to as the standard error of measurement. Because we do not know an individual's true score, we cannot calculate that individual's error score. However, using the reliability coefficient, we can estimate the standard deviation of those error scores. This value can be used to establish confidence intervals around an individual's observed score, giving an indication of the amount of error. Recall that an individual's observed score is only one possible score that might be obtained on a given test. Because we expect errors to occur, sometimes inflating a person's score and sometimes lowering the person's score, the next time the person takes the test (or completes a scale) the score is likely to be different. When the reliability of the test is high, we expect a slight difference between the scores. However, if the reliability of the test is low, the scores may differ considerably. By computing the standard error of measurement for a test, we can establish confidence intervals to estimate the range of scores within which a person's true score may fall.

The formula for calculating the standard measurement of error is shown in Equation 10.12 (Crocker & Algina, 1986).

Equation 10.11

$$\sigma_{meas} = \sigma \sqrt{1 - r_{ot}^2},$$

where

σ_{meas} = standard error of measurement,
σ = standard deviation of the observed scores, and
r_{ot}^2 = reliability coefficient.

Suppose that Jenn received a score of 88 percent on her research methods test, which has a standard deviation of 5.5 and a reliability of .78. To determine how accurate Jenn's score is, we can compute the confidence intervals around her score using Equation 10.11:

$$\sigma_{meas} = 5.5 \sqrt{1 - .78} = (5.5)(.47) = 2.6.$$

The standard error of measurement gives Jenn an indication of how much her score could change if she took the test again. To calculate confidence intervals, we simply add and subtract the standard error of measurement to and from Jenn's score. Confidence intervals within one standard deviation of the mean indicate that on repeated testing, 68 percent of the time, Jenn would receive a score within one standard deviation above and below the mean, or, in this case, a score between 85.4 percent $(88\% - 2.6)$ and 90.6 percent $(88\% + 2.6)$.

Contrast this standard error of measurement with that for Jenn's theory test. In this course, she also received a grade of 88 percent. However, the standard deviation was 3.1 and the reliability was .88. If Jenn were to take the test again, she could expect less fluctuation in her score, based on the following calculation. This result suggests that if Jenn were to take the test again, her score would likely be within 1.1 points above or below 88 percent about 68 out of 100 times.

$$\sigma_{meas} 3.1\sqrt{1 - .88} = (3.1)(3.5) = 1.1.$$

The calculation of the standard error of measurement is often used when providing students with the results of standardized tests. Sometimes rather than receiving an absolute score, students are given the range of scores in which their true score is likely to fall. Such a range is found by using the student's actual score, the standard error of measurement, and the reliability of the test. Although we have used observed scores in this example, some authors advocate the use of the predicated true score as the value around which the confidence intervals are set (Pedhazur & Schmelkin, 1991).

Generalizability Theory

CTT framed the development and testing of psychosocial and health measurement instruments throughout the twentieth century. As we learned in Chapter Nine, in CTT, the observed-score variance is partitioned into the true-score variance and the error-score variance. Reliability is defined as the ratio of true-score to observed-score variance. Earlier in this chapter, we examined different approaches to estimating reliability, each of which focused on a different source of error variance. By comparing parallel forms, we evaluate error variance attributed to different forms; for stability, we examine error variance produced by the administration of tests on different occasions; for internal consistency, we address error variance among items; and for intrarater and interrater reliability, we evaluate error variance attributed to the use of different raters or the same rater at different times. Though procedures are available to examine these different sources of error and to calculate reliability coefficients, there is no one procedure within CTT that allows the researcher to compare the relative contributions of multiple sources of error variance simultaneously (Brennan, 2001).

Cronbach (1963) recognized this problem, and in 1963, he and his colleagues introduced generalizability theory (GT). GT acknowledges that there are multiple sources of error variance in the application of instruments, and GT procedures allow the researcher to isolate and then evaluate these different sources (Brennan, 2001). Brennan (2001) has written extensively on GT and has developed analytical methods for the conduct of GT studies. The following description of GT is derived largely from his work. Using the ANOVA framework, GT procedures partition variance components into that which is due to variation in persons and that which is due to the different error components specified by the researcher. The results of a GT analysis provide an indication of the relative magnitudes of the various sources of error, and they help the researcher determine which of these sources accounts for the greatest amount of error. Using information from a GT analysis, the researcher can modify the measurement process (for example, the instrument itself, data collection procedures, or data management procedures) to reduce the identified sources of error (Brennan, 2001).

There are two types of analysis in GT. The first is called a generalizability (G) study; the second is called a decision (D) study (Brennan, 2001). The aim of the G study is to partition the variance components and estimate their magnitude. A D study uses information from the G study to evaluate outcomes associated with making selected changes in the measurement process and to identify those modifications that will result in a reduction in error variance. D studies also estimate the amount of change in error variance due to the modifications selected by the researcher for evaluation.

GT has its own set of terms, some of which we will define here. *Objects of measurement* are the participants in the research study. They are considered members of the *population*. The *universe of admissible observations* refers to the conditions of measurement. These admissible observations are the sources of error variation specified by the researcher and will differ depending on the purpose of the study. The universe of admissible observations for each study will contain at least one *facet* (source of error variance). Each facet has dimensions, called *conditions* (c). The relationships among the components for a G study are shown in Figure 10.1.

To illustrate the use of GT for estimating error variance in instrument development, suppose that Ni'Keta is interested in evaluating a newly developed nine-item scale to measure social support for people with chronic illness. Ni'Keta plans to use the instrument in a research study in which she will collect data from her participants on two occasions, three months apart. In addition to evaluating the variation

FIGURE 10.1. DIAGRAM OF THE COMPONENTS IN A G STUDY.

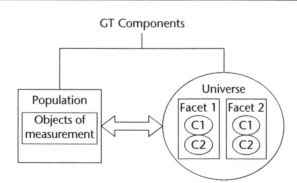

among the items, a potential source of error, she is interested in error variance due to administration of the scale on more than one occasion.

The model for her GT study consists of the participants (objects of measurement) who complete the scale on two occasions. The universe of admissible observations contains an item facet and an occasion facet. The item facet consists of nine conditions (items), and the occasion facet consists of two conditions (occasions). Ni'Keta begins with a G study, the goal of which is to divide the overall variance in the set of scores (observed-score variance) into that which is due to the object of measurement (the participants), each facet, the interaction among the object of measurement and the facets, and the residual or error variance not explained by the specified model. The variance components of most interest to Ni'Keta are those explained by the facets and their interactions with other components in the model.

A useful diagram of the variance components considered in a model such as the one Ni'Keta proposes is presented by Brennan (2001) and is shown in Figure 10.2. The decomposition of variance for the G study is shown in Equation 10.12.

Equation 10.12

$$\sigma^2(X_{pi}) = \sigma^2(p) + \sigma^2(i) + \sigma^2(o) + \sigma^2(pi) + \sigma^2(po) + \sigma^2(io) + \sigma^2(pio),$$

where

$\sigma^2(X_{pio})$ = variance of the scores over the persons in the population and the conditions in the universe of admissible observations,
$\sigma^2(p)$ = variance attributed to persons,
$\sigma^2(i)$ = variance attributed to items,
$\sigma^2(o)$ = variance attributed to occasions,
$\sigma^2(pi)$ = variance attributed to the interaction of persons and items,
$\sigma^2(po)$ = variance attributed to the interaction of persons and occasions,
$\sigma^2(io)$ = variance attributed to the interaction of items and occasions, and
$\sigma^2(pio)$ = variance attributed to the interaction of persons, items, and occasions.

To conduct the study, Ni'Keta must first collect data from participants. Her participants for this study are individuals with epilepsy, and they complete the social support scale twice, three months apart. Using ANOVA procedures, Ni'Keta is able to partition the total amount of variance in the participants' scores across both occasions into the variance components listed in Equation 10.13. Table 10.9 shows the results of the hypothetical G study conducted by Ni'Keta. The column on the left presents the different sources of variance. In this study, variance can be attributed to the participants, the items, the occasions, and the following interactions: the one between participants and items; the one between participants and occasions; the one between items and occasions; and the one among participants, items, and

FIGURE 10.2. VENN DIAGRAM FOR $P \times O \times I$ DESIGN.

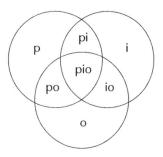

Source: R. L. Brennan, 2001, p. 56. Used by permission of Springer-Verlag.

occasions. Because it is not possible to separate out variance in the three-way interaction (participants, items, and occasions), this variance component and any remaining variance not attributed to the participants and the facets are combined together in residual or unexplained error variance. Column 2 presents the amount of variance for each component; column 3, the percentage of variance explained by each component.

In interpreting the results of the G study, we begin by examining the variance due to participants. This variance component is analogous to true-score variance in CTT and indicates differences among participants. It is generally desirable for participant variance to be relatively large when compared to other variance components. The remaining components are attributed to error. In this analysis, the largest error variance is attributed to items. Error variance of items is slightly more than three times that of the variance due to occasions, meaning that items are a greater source of variability than occasions are.

Variance components of interaction terms are more difficult to interpret, but Brennan (2001) suggests that a useful way to think of interaction is as the relative

TABLE 10.9. AMOUNT OF VARIANCE AND PERCENTAGE OF TOTAL VARIANCE FOR THE SOCIAL SUPPORT SCALE.

Source of Variation	Estimated G Study Variance Components	Percentage of Variance Explained
Participants	.455	36
Items	.332	27
Occasions	.100	8
Participant × Items	.231	18
Participant × Occasions	.020	2
Item × Occasion	.004	0
Participant × Item × Occasion + Residual Error	.115	9

standing of persons for each facet. The variance component $\sigma^2(pi)$ estimates the relative standing of persons across the items, and $\sigma^2(po)$ estimates the relative standing of persons on the two occasions. The variance component $\sigma^2(pi)$ is about ten times larger than $\sigma^2(po)$, suggesting that items are a much larger source of variance across persons than are occasions. These findings suggest that there is not much difference in the ordering of persons across the two occasions, but there is difference in the ordering of persons on the items.

Following the G study, Ni'Keta can conduct a D study. The purpose of the D study is to estimate the change in error variance when conditions within facets are changed. For example, Ni'Keta might ask what will happen to error variance if the number of items on the scale remains the same and the number of occasions is decreased to one. Ni'Keta can also calculate several coefficients that provide information about the extent to which she can generalize from this sample to a larger universe, which contains all possible conditions of the facets, without misrepresenting the data (DeVellis, 2003). The generalizability coefficient, which is analogous to the reliability coefficient in CTT, is found by dividing the variance due to persons by the sum of the variance due to persons and the relative error variance.

GT analyses, for both G and D studies, are complex and demanding. Specifications for the G study model also include making decisions about the number and nature of the facets. Before beginning a G study, the researcher must consider other factors that we have not included in the above discussion. These include defining the universe of admissible observations as *crossed* or *nested* and the facets as *random* or *fixed*. D study analysis includes the calculation of absolute error variance and relative error variance. Using this information, the researcher can calculate generalizability coefficients and the index of dependability. The analytic procedures for conducting a G study can be carried out using GENOVA (Brennan, 2001). Students interested in more detailed discussions of G theory are referred to Crick and Brennan (1983), Brennan (2001), Crocker and Algina (1986), and Shavelson and Webb (1991).

Summary

In this chapter, we have discussed different approaches to estimating reliability within CTT. These included estimates of equivalence, stability, internal consistency, and intrarater and interrater reliability. Advantages and disadvantages of the various approaches have been discussed. One major disadvantage of CTT is the inability of the researcher to estimate multiple sources of error variance at the same time. Generalizability theory, on the other hand, offers techniques to estimate multiple sources of error variance and to use the information to modify the measurement process. The specification of the model for G studies and the analytic techniques are sufficiently complex that researchers have not yet adopted them for general practice in health behavior research.

CHAPTER ELEVEN

VALIDITY

LEARNING OBJECTIVES

At the end of this chapter, the student should be able to

1. Define the term *validity*.
2. Identify the five sources of validity evidence.
3. Describe the process of assessing test content.
4. Compute a content validity index.
5. Describe the procedure of assessing response processes.
6. List the five major components of cognitive processing.
7. Describe the two primary techniques for conducting a cognitive assessment.
8. List three types of errors that can be identified through cognitive assessment.
9. Describe the procedures for assessing relationships with other variables.
10. Discuss the considerations for the criterion, construct, and multitrait-multimethod sources of validity evidence.
11. Interpret the results of the assessment for each approach.

Broadly speaking, the term *validity* refers to the legitimacy of an instrument—that is, does it measure what it purports to measure? (See Nunnally & Bernstein, 1994.) Validity is not a characteristic of an instrument itself. It is, rather, the degree of support obtained for the interpretations of scores on an instrument when the instrument is used for its intended purpose (American Educational Research Association, American Psychological Association, and National Council on Measurement in Education, 1999). Thus, it is not the instrument that is validated; it is the interpretation of scores and actions based on those scores that is validated (Messick, 1989). Consider, for example, an achievement test designed to assess the math skills of sixth-grade students. A cursory review of the test shows items assessing the student's ability to add, subtract, multiply, and divide. Because the items assess math concepts that have been taught to sixth-grade students, the results of the test provide a valid indication of the math skills of these students. The results of the test can be used to determine whether the students have successfully mastered the content of one unit before moving on to the next unit. Although the items assess math concepts, if the same test were given to first-grade students, the results would not be valid, because we would not expect the average first-grade student to understand these higher-level math concepts. And these latter results could not be used to document successful mastery of math concepts by first-grade students. Likewise, a scale designed to measure health behaviors of adolescents with chronic illnesses might be a valid measure for adolescents with diabetes, but not a valid measure of health behaviors of adolescents free of chronic health problems.

Because validity is a function of inferences from scores on an instrument, it is important to specify the intended purpose of the instrument, the intended population for which it will be used, and the conditions under which inferences can be made. For the development of a scale, these specifications consist of a complete description of the construct, including its conceptual basis and dimensions. Embedded within this description are the results of the concept analysis, which specify the theoretical definition of the construct, its defining characteristics, the characteristics that distinguish it from other constructs, and proposed relationships to other constructs. The specifications also include descriptions of the instrument, the calculation of scores, the interpretation of scores, and the conditions under which the scale is to be used. In Chapter Seven, we provided a description of the construct of outcome expectations for healthy eating. To begin a validity assessment of the OE scale, we would also need to specify how the instrument is to be used, the population for which the instrument is intended, and the conditions under which inferences can be made. We might specify that the OE for healthy eating scale be designed as a research instrument to assess the possible outcomes that older men and women associate with eating a healthy diet. Based on the conceptual framework, we might also state that the scale can be used in studies to predict eating behaviors.

Test validation is the process of gathering evidence to support the interpretation of scores and subsequent decisions based on those scores (American Educational Research Association et al., 1999; Messick, 1989). Both theoretical and empirical evidence is used in the validation process (Messick, 1989). That is, the developer must demonstrate, through the use of theory and empirical evidence, that the interpretation and use of scores are correct and are built on sound science. Of necessity, the validation process involves designing studies and collecting data to demonstrate that the instrument functions in the way in which it was designed to function. Once in use, an instrument is continually assessed to gather supporting evidence, but the accumulation of support takes time. Sometimes the performance of the instrument under different conditions suggests that changes are needed in the instrument or in its use. Take, for example, a scale developed to measure depressive symptoms in adults with chronic illnesses. This scale might function as intended for men and women with diabetes, but lack validity evidence when used for adults with HIV. Data obtained from men and women with HIV might provide information that would help the researcher to modify the scale for use with these adults. Because gathering validity evidence is a continual process, validity is never fully established, but is rather considered a matter of degree based on the amount and kind of accrued evidence (American Educational Research Association et al., 1999).

During the twentieth century, psychometricians proposed different approaches to test validation. These approaches were treated as separate forms of validity, and each was given a name. *Content validity* is defined as the assessment of the correspondence between the items composing the instrument and the content domain from which the items are selected. *Criterion-related validity* is the assessment of the correspondence between the scores on the instrument and scores on selected outcome variables. And *construct validity* is the assessment of the correspondence between scores on the instrument and scores on similar or different constructs. Content validity has a similar, but less rigorous, form known as *face validity*. Criterion-related validity has subcategories called *predictive* and *concurrent validity;* construct validity has the subcategories of *convergent, discriminant,* and *known group validity*. Results obtained from factor analysis are also used to determine construct validity. Over the years, researchers have applied these types of validity differently, which has led to confusion about the meaning of some forms of validity and the procedures for testing them.

To help clarify the conceptualization of validity, Messick (1989) proposed that validity is a unitary concept that depends on the accrual of evidence from different sources (Messick, 1989; American Educational Research Association et al., 1999). In Messick's model, the traditional types of validity—content, criterion, and construct— are considered to be sources of validity evidence and not types of validity. Though some have adopted Messick's conceptualization of validity (American Educational Research Association et al., 1999), in general, researchers have been reluctant to use the new terminology in place of the old. For this reason, we include both the new and the old terminology in the discussion below and present a comparison of the two in Table 11.1.

TABLE 11.1. NEW AND OLD TERMINOLOGY FOR VALIDITY.

New	Old
Sources of Validity Evidence	**Types of Validity**
Evidence based on test content	Content validity
Evidence based on response processes	Cognitive assessment
Evidence based on relations with other variables	Criterion validity Construct validity Multitrait-multimethod matrix
Evidence based on internal structure	Factor analysis Item response theory
Evidence based on consequences of testing	None

Source: Items in the new terminology column are drawn from American Educational Research Association et al., 1999.

The latest standards for education and psychological testing (American Educational Research Association et al., 1999) list five sources of validity evidence. These are

- Test content
- Response processes
- Relations to other variables
- Internal structure
- Consequences of testing

In this chapter, we discuss the first three concepts—test content, response processes, and relations to other variables—and in Chapters Twelve and Thirteen, we will discuss two procedures for assessing the internal structures of scales.

Test Content

Test content, more commonly referred to as content validity, is the first source of validity evidence that is gathered. The primary purpose of gathering content-validity evidence is to confirm that the items written for the instrument adequately represent the construct. Ideally, items written for a scale measure the construct as defined in the theoretical definition. Scale items can also be written to measure dimensions of the construct. The researcher can significantly improve the chances of an adequate representation of items by (1) using a content-by-dimension matrix to identify the types of items that should be included in the instrument, (2) developing a thoughtful item-writing plan, and (3) carefully implementing the item-writing procedures. For example, a researcher who intends to measure the three dimensions of OE would include a sufficient number of items to measure the self-evaluative, social, and physical dimensions of OE. A scale to measure social support would likely include items related to family, friends, and perhaps coworkers.

The use of a carefully specified plan including the table of test specifications, or matrix, documents the direct link between the theoretical definition of content domain and the items. This documentation can serve as a source of validity evidence and is called *a priori content validity* (Waltz, Strickland, & Lenz, 1991). Though a careful item-writing process provides some evidence for validity, a priori content validity fails to completely answer the question, Do the items themselves adequately measure the construct or content domain? To answer this question, additional review by content experts, measurement specialists, and potential respondents is generally necessary.

Procedures

The content validity process we describe here is similar to the process used to assess the content validity of knowledge tests. We described that procedure in Chapter Five. In the present discussion, we focus on the use of the procedure for assessing the content validity of scales.

The content validity process begins with selecting content and measurement experts to evaluate the instrument and the individual items. The group of experts should include individuals who know the content area well and experts in measurement. The content experts are able to evaluate the extent to which the items adequately measure the content domain or scale dimensions. Measurement experts might not be able to adequately judge the content of the items, but they generally have more experience than the content experts in item development and can more readily identify problematic item structure (for example, jargon or double-barreled items).

The second step in the process is to develop the materials for the assessment. To conduct an adequate assessment, the expert reviewers will need (1) written instructions explaining how to evaluate the scale; (2) an overview of the construct, including the theoretical definition and examples; (3) a description of the scale, including number of items, scoring, and reverse-coded items; (4) a copy of the actual scale that a participant would complete; and (5) an evaluation form for rating items. Exhibit 11.1 presents the materials for the assessment of the OE for healthy eating scale.

To conduct a content validity assessment, experts review each item separately and then review the overall scale. Usually experts are asked to make two kinds of judgments. They are asked to rate (1) the extent to which each item adequately reflects the theoretical definition of the construct for a scale or the content domain and (2) the extent to which the entire set of items represents the construct or content domain. A common procedure is to ask experts to rate each item on its degree of relevance.

EXHIBIT 11.1. EXAMPLE OF MATERIALS FOR CONDUCTING A CONTENT VALIDITY ASSESSMENT.

Instructions for the Content Experts

Thank you for agreeing to review and evaluate the scale we have developed for our study, the Healthy Lifestyle Program. You were selected for this task because of your interest and expertise in the development of scales to measure outcome expectations.

At this time we need your assistance in assessing the content validity of our new scale to measure outcome expectations for healthy eating among older adults. This task involves rating the relevancy of each item to the concept of outcome expectations.

The following information is included:

1. Description of the conceptual framework for scale development
2. Description of the scale
3. Form for rating item-relevancy

The procedure for this task is

1. Read the description of the theoretical basis of scale development.
2. Using the rating form, rate each item as to its degree of relevance in measuring the concept of outcome expectations.
3. Note whether items are appropriate to measure healthy eating.
4. Make any suggestions you may have for the addition or deletion of items or for changes in the wording of items on the form itself.
5. Evaluate the instructions for the scale.
6. Evaluate the format of the scale.

Conceptual Framework for Scale Development

Bandura's social cognitive theory formed the theoretical basis for the development of the instrument to measure outcome expectations related to healthy eating. Bandura (1997) defines outcome expectations as the outcomes that one expects to occur if he or she performs a specific behavior. For example, one individual might expect that he would fall off a horse and get injured if he were to attempt to ride a horse. Another person might expect that she would be tired all the time if she exercised three times per week, whereas her friend might expect that she would prevent diseases such as stroke if she exercised. Bandura notes that outcome expectations have a powerful influence on behavior. People who expect more positive outcomes associated with behaviors are more likely to perform the behaviors, whereas those who associate negative outcomes with specific behaviors are less likely to perform the behaviors.

Description of the Scale

For this scale we are interested in the behavior of eating a healthy diet among older men and women. We are interested in measuring the outcomes older adults expect if they eat a low-fat diet high in fruits and vegetables. Once developed and tested, the scale will be used in research studies to assess the role of outcome expectations in the eating behaviors.

This scale is composed of twelve items. Each item is rated on a four-point scale from (1) <u>strongly disagree</u> to (4) <u>strongly agree</u>. Responses to each item are summed to yield a total score. Total scores range from 12 to 48; higher scores indicate more positive outcome expectations related to eating a healthy diet.

Relevancy Rating Form

Instructions: Please use the following form to rate the relevancy of each item to the concept of outcome expectations as defined by Bandura. Please read each item carefully; then rate each item on the four-point scale in terms of how relevant you believe it is in measuring the concept of outcome expectations.

1 = not relevant
2 = somewhat relevant
3 = quite relevant
4 = very relevant

1.	If you eat a healthy diet, you will have more energy.	1	2	3	4
2.	If you eat a healthy diet, you feel better about yourself.	1	2	3	4
3.	If you eat a healthy diet, you will live longer.	1	2	3	4
4.	If you eat a healthy diet, your best friends will approve.	1	2	3	4
5.	If you eat a healthy diet, your friends will be proud of you.	1	2	3	4
6.	If you eat a healthy diet, you will control your weight.	1	2	3	4
7.	If you eat a healthy diet, you will feel proud of yourself.	1	2	3	4
8.	If you eat a healthy diet, you will be less likely to have a stroke.	1	2	3	4
9.	If you eat a healthy diet, you will feel more responsible.	1	2	3	4
10.	If you eat a healthy diet, you will feel you are doing the right thing.	1	2	3	4
11.	If you eat a healthy diet, your doctor will approve.	1	2	3	4
12.	If you eat a healthy diet, your close relatives will approve.	1	2	3	4

Waltz, Strickland, and Lenz (1991) suggest a four-point rating scale with 1 = *not relevant*, 2 = *somewhat relevant*, 3 = *quite relevant*, and 4 = *very relevant*. Lynn (1986) also suggests a four-point rating scale, with 1 = *not relevant*; 2 = *unable to assess relevance without item revision, or item is in need of such revision that it would no longer be relevant*; 3 = *relevant but needs minor alteration*; and 4 = *very relevant and succinct*.

Experts evaluate the wording of each item and the response format and examine items for cultural or gender bias. They also review other aspects of the scale, including the clarity of instructions and the formatting, and assess the degree to which the overall set of items represents the construct or content domain. The experts are then asked to suggest revisions, including the addition and deletion of items. If the researcher has developed items to measure more than one dimension of a scale, the evaluation can include asking experts to rate each item on its relevance to a particular dimension. For example, with the OE for healthy eating scale, the researcher might ask the experts, first, to rate each item as a measure of OE and then to rate each item according to its degree of fit with the self-evaluative, social, or physical dimension. The researcher might also want to know whether the items are adequate reflections of a healthy diet.

Content Validity Index

Following the evaluation, the researcher collects the rating forms and summarizes the data. If a rating scale is used, a content validity index (CVI) can be calculated. There are several ways to calculate a CVI. One way, suggested by Waltz, Strickland, and Lenz (1991), requires two experts, called judges. This approach calculates an overall percentage of agreement between the judges. To use this approach, the researcher records the number of items both judges rate as either a 3 (quite relevant) or a 4 (very relevant). The number of items both judges rate as a 3 or 4 is divided by the total number of items. Suppose that both judges rated the same ten items as 3 or 4 on the twelve-item OE for healthy eating scale. One judge rated OE6 as 2 and the other rated the same item as 3. One judge rated OE9 as 1 and the other rated it as 3. To compute a CVI, the number of items both judges rate as a 3 or 4 (ten) is divided by the total number of items (twelve) as follows:

$$\frac{10}{12} = .83.$$

The CVI for this set of items, computed from ratings by these two judges, is .83. This approach provides a CVI for the entire instrument.

If a researcher is using more than two experts (which is recommended), a CVI can be calculated by first determining the percentage of items that are rated as 3 or 4 for each expert. These percentages are summed and divided by the number of experts to determine the content validity for the entire scale. If we had five experts and three of them rated 92 percent of the items as either 3 or 4 and two rated all the items (100 percent) as either 3 or 4, then

Equation 11.1

$$CVI = \frac{\sum \%}{N},$$

$$CVI = \frac{3 \times 92\% + 2 \times 100\%}{5}, \text{ and}$$

$$= \frac{476\%}{5} = 95\%.$$

To determine which items are problematic, the researcher can compute CVIs for individual items. To do so, the researcher calculates the percentage of experts who rate an item as quite relevant or very relevant. Suppose we had five experts, and two of them rated OE3 as not relevant (1), one rated it as somewhat relevant (2), and two rated it as quite relevant (4). Thus:

$$CVI = \frac{2}{5} \times 100 = 40\%.$$

The CVI for each item—or for the total scale—can range from 0 to 1. The usual recommendation is that the CVI should be at least .90 (Waltz, Strickland, & Lenz, 1991) for the entire instrument and also for the individual items. Following the recommendations of the experts, the researcher can make improvements in items. Rewording a problematic item might make it more consistent with the meaning of the construct or the content domain, and deleting problematic items will likely improve the overall CVI.

After the items are revised, they can be reevaluated by the same group of experts. If extensive revisions are necessary, the researcher might request another review of all the items, either by the same experts or by a new group of experts. Following this evaluation, a new CVI is calculated. If the CVI is .90 or greater, the researcher can continue the evaluation process using additional tests of reliability and validity. An unacceptable CVI after a second evaluation suggests that the entire developmental process must be reevaluated before the researcher proceeds to additional psychometric testing.

Despite the appeal of this method of evaluating scale content, expert judgment is not infallible. Sometimes, experts may believe that an item is an adequate measure of a construct, but when the item is examined using other procedures, it is found to be flawed. Thus, though the assessment of test content is one source of validity information, it cannot be the only source.

Face Validity

Content validity has struggled for many years to gain full status as a legitimate form of validity assessment. One of the reasons is that some researchers confuse content validity with face validity. Face validity consists of a cursory review of an instrument and items to determine whether they seem to measure what the developer claims they measure. Face validity involves a simple reading of the items and a judgment about the correspondence between the items and the definition of the construct or content domain. Face validity lacks the rigor of a content validity assessment because it does not include a rating for each item and a calculation of a validity index. The student should be aware that although some authors claim that they have conducted a content validity assessment, a careful reading of the report or article may reveal a process that is more similar to face validity than it is to content validity.

Response Processes

A second source of validity evidence is obtained by evaluating responses of participants to individual items on an instrument. Cognitive assessment is one method designed to assess how individuals understand and respond to items (Tourangeau & Rasinski, 1988). The procedures for a cognitive assessment were originally developed to evaluate survey items, but the process can be applied easily to the evaluation of items developed for scales or achievement tests. Cognitive assessment is based on the idea that an individual uses a series of cognitive processes to answer items. By understanding how people answer specific items, the researcher can determine whether an item is being answered in the way in which it was intended to be answered or whether alternative interpretations are being used to respond to the item. The researcher can also determine how people make decisions about how to answer an item. The purpose of cognitive assessment is to discover how respondents interpret items and whether their interpretations of the items are similar to those of the instrument developer (Sudman, Bradburn, & Schwarz, 1996). Using this approach and the right type of probes, the researcher can also determine the presence of response sets such as social desirability. Armed with this information, the researcher can modify items to clarify meaning and, in turn, reduce respondent error.

Tourangeau and Rasinski (1988) delineate five major components of the cognitive process used to answer questionnaire items: comprehension, interpretation, recall, judgment, and response. To respond to an item, a participant must first comprehend what is being requested. The participant must then interpret the request and decide how to respond to it. In formulating a response, the participant must retrieve information from memory. When the information has been retrieved, the participant must decide what information to provide to answer the item. Here, the participant must decide whether his or her memory has been searched sufficiently to answer the item, whether the selected response is good enough, and whether the response is acceptable. Based on the circumstances in which the data are being collected, response bias might be a factor in making the final decision about how to answer an item. Finally, the participant must provide an answer in the format requested or decide on another format if he or she believes that the required format is inadequate.

For example, if a female participant is asked how often she exercised last week, she must first decide what activities constitute exercise. Does exercise include gardening or is the researcher only interested in planned periods of exercise such as running or swimming? After she makes a decision about what exercise is, she must search her memory to determine how many times in the past week she has exercised. If she runs on a regular basis, she might respond by giving the average number of times she runs each week. If she wants to give a more exact answer, she might spend a few minutes to determine the exact number of days on which she ran. Finally, she must write down a response in the format requested. In this case, the researcher is interested in the number of times the respondent has exercised in the past week. For our runner, who has determined that the researcher is interested in planned periods of exercise, a response of 3 might be appropriate. A woman who does not exercise might be reluctant to say so and might give a number greater than 0, displaying a social-desirability response set. A woman who believes that the researcher is interested in both planned and unplanned periods of exercise, including housework and gardening, might give an answer of 10, reflecting these latter activities as well as planned activities such as yoga. The researcher might be unaware of the different interpretations made by various participants of what seems to be a fairly simple item on the questionnaire.

Procedures

As with the content validity process, cognitive assessment begins with developing a plan for the assessment. The plan should include the items to be assessed, the number of participants, the approach (thinking aloud or verbal probes), and materials for recording information. Once the plan is developed, participants are recruited into the study. Usually ten to twelve people selected from the population of interest are included in the assessment. The researcher meets with each person individually to conduct the assessment, which can take one to two hours to complete, depending on the number of items assessed.

Think Aloud. There are two primary approaches for conducting a cognitive assessment: the think-aloud method and the verbal-probe method. In the think-aloud method, the researcher asks the respondents to think aloud as they respond to the item. The researcher asks the respondents to tell him or her what they are thinking as they construct an answer to the question. The researcher records such statements from a sample of participants and uses this information to determine whether the respondents understand the item, the factors related to the ways respondents answered, and the ways in which the respondents generated the answer.

For example, thinking aloud, one of the participants in the exercise study might say the following when asked if she exercised last week: "Well, I did not go running. I don't have anyone around to play basketball with, and I don't belong to a baseball team, although we have a corporate team. I don't belong to a gym or one of those spas. I can't afford it. I used to run, but don't any more, so I guess the answer would be no."

In responding to the item, the participant seemed to interpret the word *exercise* to mean planned exercise. Team sports and aerobic activities would probably be included in her definition if she were forced to define exercise. She did not seem to think of strength or flexibility activities or household activities as exercise. She was able to respond in the correct manner (*yes* or *no*), but it is unclear whether she searched her memory for each day of the week. It seems that after she decided that only planned aerobic activities and team sports were defined as exercise, the decision was easy for her, because she had engaged in none of these in the preceding week.

Despite its appeal, participants often find the think-aloud method difficult. The cognitive processes used to respond to items occur in rapid succession. The technique requires that respondents slow down the process and think through each of the steps—comprehension, interpretation, recall, judgment, and response—and describe these processes to the researcher. Participants often find it hard to describe the processes they are using in sufficient detail for the researcher to obtain useful information. If this method is used, the researcher should provide some practice items that are not related to the survey to help the respondent learn the technique. In addition to the method's difficulty for some respondents, it is not effective when the researcher is asking about sensitive topics, including sexual behavior and drug use. Consider, for example, asking a respondent to think aloud while constructing a response to this question: When was the last time you used a condom?

Verbal Probe. In the verbal-probe method, the researcher constructs questions about the item ahead of time. These questions, called probes, are used to gather information about the way the respondent processed the question. The researcher then asks the respondent to answer each question as it is asked. Following the response, the researcher then asks the respondent questions about the way the item was processed and the way the response was selected. By planning ahead, the researcher can use the same probes for all the respondents. For example, the researcher can ask all the respondents whether they understood certain terms or ask them to tell him or her what certain terms meant to them. The researcher can also ask how they determined how many times they had done something in the past week or month or year and can also determine whether they used different methods to calculate their responses. Exhibit 11.2 presents an example of verbal probes for a set of items about exercise.

Evaluation

The descriptive data obtained from the cognitive assessment are used to make decisions about the items and any modifications that might be necessary. A well-conducted cognitive assessment can provide the researcher with valuable information about the construction of individual items. Problems and processes that can be identified through this method include

- Terms that are not understood by or that have different meanings for the respondents
- Vagueness or ambiguity in the questions themselves
- Items that participants respond to without knowing their content
- Difficulty in recalling information for the time frame provided
- Problems with the response choices
- Processes used to calculate events
- Processes used to recall information
- Factors associated with making the final responses

Using the cognitive-assessment approach and the right type of probes, the researcher can also determine the presence of response sets or the presence of overlapping concepts. For example, a researcher who is developing a scale to measure depression might find that some symptoms commonly associated with depression (for example, fatigue and insomnia) have other reasons besides depression. If items related to fatigue and insomnia are included on the depression scale, a person having difficulty sleeping during the nights before his or her wedding may be inaccurately

EXHIBIT 11.2. EXAMPLE OF VERBAL PROBES USED IN AN ASSESSMENT.

In this cognitive assessment, the researcher is interested in learning how people interpret the word *exercise.* The researcher also wants to know how people calculate the number of times that they exercise and how they perceive the time frames of *currently* and the *past week.*

Question 1: Do you currently exercise?

Questions About the Term *Exercise*
- What types of exercise do you know about?
- What came to your mind when you were asked about exercise?
- Tell me what the term ***exercise*** means to you.
- Does exercise include aerobic activities such as running?
- If so, which ones would you include?
- Does exercise include strength activities such as weight lifting?
- If so, are there others that you would include?
- Does exercise include stretching and flexibility exercises such as yoga?
- If so, which others would you include?
- Does exercise include household chores that require movement, such as vacuuming?
- If so, which others would you include?
- Are there any that you can think of that you would not include?

- Does exercise include outside chores that require movement, such as mowing the lawn?
- If so, which others would you include?
- Are there any that you can think of that you would not include?
- Are there any other activities you can think of that we did not talk about?

Questions About the Term *Currently*
- What does the word *currently* mean to you?
- What time frame would it include?
- Would the past week be currently?
- Would the past year be currently?
- How far back would currently go?

Question 2: How many times in the past week did you exercise?

Question About the Term *Exercise*
- What activities did you include for exercise?

Question About the Term *How Many Times*
- Tell me how you counted the number of times that you exercised during the past week.

Questions About the Term *Past Week*
- What does the term *past week* mean to you?
- What days (dates) did you consider for determining the past week?
- How far back did you go?

---

diagnosed with depression. The cognitive-assessment method is informally used when students give feedback to the instructor after taking a test. Students often state that their interpretation of an item or one of the responses was different from the interpretation intended by the instructor who developed the test. Such feedback may benefit students who can convince the instructor of their arguments and receive credit for their responses. The wise instructor will take these comments into consideration and revise questionable test items before using them with future classes of students. Careful rewording of an item or response choices in light of the results of a cognitive assessment can reduce the possibility of error due to a poor item.

Relationships to Other Variables

A third way to obtain evidence for validity is to examine the relationship between the construct measured by the new scale and other constructs. As shown in Table 11.1, the approaches to examining relationships have traditionally been labeled (1) *criterion validity*, (2) *construct validity*, and (3) *multitrait-multimethod validity*. Criterion validity is composed of two subtypes, concurrent validity and predictive validity, both of which include the comparison of the new scale to a criterion variable. For construct validity, theory and previous research findings are used to select constructs and to create hypotheses of relationships between the construct measured by the new scale and theoretically related constructs. The multitrait-multimethod procedure allows the researcher to examine relationships between the same and different constructs measured using at least two different methods. In each case, the determination of validity is based on the extent to which the constructs are correlated in the predicted direction.

Criterion Validity

Criterion validity was first proposed by Cronbach and Meehl (1955). As the name implies, a criterion is used in validity assessment. A criterion is a variable that one wishes to predict by using information from another variable, called a predictor variable (Pedhazur & Schmelkin, 1991). A criterion can be an outcome such as success in college, job satisfaction, adherence to a treatment regimen, or posttraumatic stress disorder. A criterion can also be an established instrument measuring the same construct as the new scale. In criterion validity, the researcher attempts to show that scores on the criterion variable can be determined from scores on the predictor variable. When the researcher is testing a new scale, the new instrument assumes the role of the predictor variable. Thus, if the scores on the new scale predict the scores on the criterion as expected, evidence exists to support the validity of the new scale.

There are many examples of relationships between criterion and predictor variables in our daily lives. Perhaps the most common example of criterion validity is the use of Scholastic Aptitude Test (SAT) scores to predict success in college. College admission committees review SAT scores because students who score high on the SAT also tend to have higher college grade point averages, which are indicators of college success. Students who successfully complete a course of study (for example, a master's degree program in public health) are more likely to be successful in their careers than those who do not. Likewise, employers may use some testing procedures to select job applicants who possess the necessary skills for a position. In each case, scores on the predictor variables (SAT, course of study, job test) are used to predict an outcome (college, career, or employment success).

When the predictor and criterion variables are measured at about the same time, the term *concurrent validity* is used. The comparison between a new instrument and an established instrument, sometimes called the *gold standard*, is a good example. Body fat measured using hydrostatic weighing could be considered the criterion variable for the assessment of body fat by measuring skin fold thickness (predictor). Criterion validity is called predictive validity when the assessment of the predictor variable precedes that of the criterion variable. In this approach, data for the predictor variable are collected first and are used to predict scores on the criterion, for which data are collected some time later. The best example of predictive validity is the use of scores from the SAT to predict college success. Another example is one's score on a driving test (predictor) and the number and type of driving violations recorded one year later.

When using criterion validity to assess a new scale, the developer begins by identifying a suitable criterion for the new measure. The criterion can be an outcome predicted from scores on the new scale or an established instrument measuring the same construct as the new measure. For example, a new scale designed to measure depression could be compared to the clinician's psychological assessment, considered the gold standard. To conduct the assessment, an instrument to measure the criterion must exist and must show evidence that it is a reliable and valid measure of the criterion. Next, the researcher selects a sample of participants representing those for whom the instrument will ultimately be used. If concurrent validity is being assessed, both measures (the new scale and the criterion) are completed by the participants at the same time (or within a short period of time). If predictive validity is being assessed, data are obtained from the new scale before being obtained from the criterion.

Researchers are likely to use the Pearson product moment correlation coefficient to assess the relationship between the predictor and criterion variables that are continuous and cross-tabulations for variables that are dichotomous. The correlation coefficient is sometimes referred to as the validity coefficient. The square of the validity coefficient is called the coefficient of determination.

There are no standard guidelines for determining how strong a correlation must be for the researcher to declare that criterion validity evidence exists. To some extent it depends on the constructs and the measures under evaluation. Measures of the same construct would be expected to have relatively high correlations, some more than others. For example, if a researcher developed a new instrument to measure body temperature, a nearly perfect correlation between readings from the new instrument and from a mercury thermometer would be expected. Likewise, readings from new instruments to measure other body attributes, such as weight and blood pressure, would be expected to be strongly correlated with readings from the gold standard for each of these measures. The correlations between new instruments measuring psychosocial constructs, such as depression, self-esteem, and self-efficacy, and established measures of these constructs are likely to show weaker correlations ranging perhaps from .6 to .8.

When predictive validity is assessed over a short time period, correlations ranging from .4 to .7 may be acceptable. However, longer time periods between the measures of the predictor and the criterion are likely to demonstrate small to moderate correlations (that is, .3 to .5.). Low correlations (that is, <.2), even if they are statistically significant, may not provide the evidence needed to support a given use of the new measure for its intended purpose. Likewise, correlations that are lower than expected without explanation lead the researcher to question whether or not the new instrument measures what it purports to measure or can be used for its intended purpose. For example, a correlation of .8 between a new instrument for measuring blood pressure and the gold standard would not be considered adequate. Whatever the value of the validity coefficient, it is the responsibility of the researcher to determine whether or not the assessment provides evidence for validity and to provide the rationale for doing so.

Suppose that Carley, a health educator working with adolescents who are HIV-positive, is concerned that many of them do not take their antiretroviral medications (ARTs) as instructed. By not taking their medications consistently, they increase their risk of developing resistant strains of HIV. Carley has developed a scale to assess readiness to take HIV medications and would like to assess the scale for criterion validity. Because the scale will be used to assess readiness to take medications, she selects actual medication adherence as the criterion variable. She expects that if the scale really measures readiness to take antiretroviral medications consistently, it should be correlated with actual adherence, meaning that teens who score high on the readiness scale (that is, they demonstrate the skills and motivation to take their medications regularly) will also take their medicines as instructed.

To test the hypothesis, she asks a sample of adolescents to complete the readiness scale. Total scores on the readiness scale range from 0 to 10; higher scores correspond to more readiness to begin a medication regimen. She then asks these adolescents to use a diary for three months to record the days and times when they take their medications. At the end of three months, she examines the association between the scores on the readiness scale and the percentage of medication doses taken on time. Hypothetical data for the results of such a study are displayed in Table 11.2. The correlation between the scores on the readiness scale and the percentage of medications taken correctly is .756, which is statistically significant ($p = .011$). This correlation indicates that as readiness scores increase, so do the percentages of doses taken on time. Although this is not a perfect correlation, on the average, adolescents who score high on the readiness test are also those who are more likely to take their medications correctly. The scatterplot in Figure 11.1 shows that those who score 7 and higher on the readiness test have a higher average percentage of adherence than those who score lower.

Based on this information, Carley concludes that the assessment provides evidence for using the readiness scale to help select those adolescents who are ready to assume responsibility for medication taking. Remember that *validity* refers to the interpretation of the scores for a given population and not of the instrument itself. Thus, health educators and others cannot use this scale without further testing to assess readiness for antiretroviral medication taking among adults or people with other health conditions.

TABLE 11.2. HYPOTHETICAL SCORES OF PARTICIPANTS ON A READI-NESS SCALE AND PERCENTAGE OF DOSES TAKEN CORRECTLY.

Participant ID	Readiness Score	Adherence Percentage
1	6	90
2	3	60
3	1	30
4	8	95
5	7	100
6	6	85
7	7	80
8	4	30
9	9	90
10	8	60
Mean	5.9	72

FIGURE 11.1. SPSS PRINTOUT OF SCATTERPLOT SHOWING THE RELATIONSHIP BETWEEN READINESS SCORES AND MEDICATION ADHERENCE FOR A HYPOTHETICAL SET OF DATA.

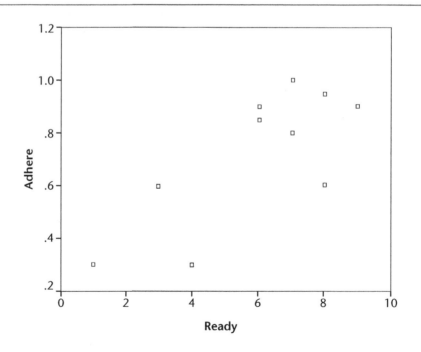

Construct Validity

For many years, criterion validity was the mainstay of validity assessment. Researchers recognized, however, that for many constructs for which they were developing measures, there were no suitable criteria for comparison. This was particularly true for psychological constructs that measured internal processes such as anxiety and ego strength (Cronbach & Meehl, 1955). To overcome this shortcoming, Cronbach and Meehl proposed an approach called construct validity. They noted that even though many constructs do not have criteria to predict, constructs rarely stand alone. Most are embedded within a network of constructs held together with propositional statements. These networks or theories (other names include *conceptual* or *theoretical frameworks* and *nomological networks*) provide explanations of constructs including their relationships with other constructs. Figure 11.2 shows an example of such a network for the construct of self-efficacy. This model shows that there are four sources of self-efficacy: previous performance, vicarious experience, verbal persuasion, and affective state. It also depicts the propositions that people who are highly self-efficacious are likely to hold more positive expectations associated with a behavior and to have more specific goals for performance and are more likely to perform the behavior.

Cronbach and Meehl (1955) reasoned that if an instrument measured what it was intended to measure, its relationships with other constructs would conform to the relationships dictated by the theory. To examine relationships, the researcher selects one or more constructs that are theoretically related to the construct measured by the new scale. The researcher can select those that are expected to show a positive relationship, a negative relationship, or no relationship with the construct measured by the new

FIGURE 11.2. HYPOTHESIZED RELATIONSHIPS AMONG VARIABLES WITHIN SOCIAL COGNITIVE THEORY.

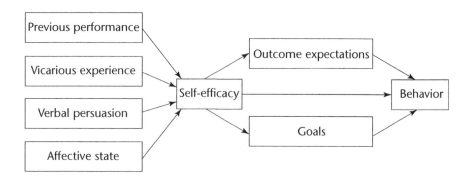

instrument. Hypotheses are generated and tested for each relationship and the results are compared to the hypothesized relationships. Evidence for validity is obtained when the hypothesized relationships are supported.

Suppose a researcher develops a new scale to measure self-efficacy to take anti-retroviral medications (medication self-efficacy). To test for construct validity, the researcher uses self-efficacy theory (Figure 11.3) to hypothesize that medication self-efficacy is positively related to OE for medication taking, positively related to social support (a measure of verbal persuasion), negatively related to difficult life circumstances, and not related to age. According to the theory (Bandura, 1997), individuals who display high levels of self-efficacy for a particular behavior report more positive outcomes associated with that behavior (OE). Moreover, people who are in supportive situations are more likely to develop self-efficacy. This relationship suggests that those living under challenging circumstances (that is, difficult life circumstances) may have lower levels of support and thus less self-efficacy. Bandura (1997) points out that self-efficacy is behavior-specific and therefore the researcher believes that age should not be related to self-efficacy. The relationships and the direction—positive, negative, or neutral—that will be tested are displayed in Figure 11.3.

To conduct the test of the hypotheses, the researcher asks participants to complete the new medication self-efficacy scale and measures to assess OE, social support, and difficult life circumstances. Background information, including age, is also collected. It is important to note that the instruments selected to measure OE, social support, and difficult life circumstances should be existing measures that have evidence of reliability and validity. Statistical tests are conducted to determine the degree to which the scores on the new instrument are correlated with age and with the scores on OE, social support, and difficult life circumstances. The results of the statistical tests for the medication self-efficacy scale are presented in Table 11.3. As anticipated, self-efficacy is positively correlated with OE ($r = .44$) and social support ($r = .36$), and it is negatively

FIGURE 11.3. HYPOTHESIZED RELATIONSHIPS AMONG VARIABLES TO BE EXAMINED.

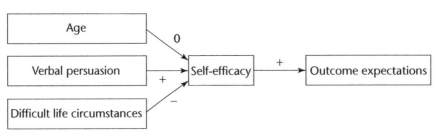

correlated with difficult life circumstances ($r = -.38$) and not correlated with age ($r = .02$). The hypotheses are supported, indicating that the new instrument behaves as expected according to theory. Thus, there is support for the belief that the scores on the new instrument can be used to measure medication self-efficacy.

Another way to assess construct validity is to examine differences between groups using the *known-groups approach*. In this approach, participants are selected based on their membership in one of two or more groups that are expected to differ on the construct of interest. The researcher tests the hypothesis that one group of participants will score higher (or lower) on the new scale than another group of participants. For example, with the medication self-efficacy scale, the researcher could collect data from participants on their current medication-taking behaviors (adherence). Based on social cognitive theory, it is expected that individuals who take their medications consistently (known group 1) would have a higher mean score on the self-efficacy scale than participants who frequently miss doses of medication (known group 2). ANOVA or the t test is generally used to assess the difference between the mean scale scores of the two groups. Table 11.4 presents the results of a test of the hypothesis that the participants who took 90 percent or more of their medication doses within the past month (known group 1) had a higher mean self-efficacy score than those who took less than 90 percent of the required doses (known group 2). The results show that the mean scores differ significantly between the two groups, providing support for construct validity.

A third way to assess construct validity is to examine the way scores on the instrument change over time. Again, theory serves as the basis for the selection of variables and hypotheses for the test. Under certain conditions, we might expect to see changes in scores on the new instrument. For example, if Carley, the health educator, developed a medication program to increase the adolescents' confidence in taking their antiretroviral medications, she would expect to see scores on the self-efficacy instrument

TABLE 11.3. CORRELATION COEFFICIENTS FOR RELATIONSHIPS BETWEEN SELF-EFFICACY AND OUTCOME EXPECTATIONS, SOCIAL SUPPORT, DIFFICULT LIFE CIRCUMSTANCES, AND AGE.

	Self-Efficacy	
	r	*p*
Outcome expectations	.44	.000
Social support	.36	.000
Difficult life circumstances	−.38	.000
Age	.02	.652

TABLE 11.4. SPSS PRINTOUT OF ANOVA FOR HYPOTHETICAL DATA COMPARING DIFFERENCES BETWEEN TWO GROUPS ON A SELF-EFFICACY SCALE.

ANOVA

EFFICACY

	Sum of Squares	df	Mean Square	F	Sig.
Between Groups	26242.139	1	26242.139	15.727	.000
Within Groups	518947.9	311	1668.643		
Total	545190.1	312			

increase after the program. She might expect, for example, that adolescents who attended the program would score higher on the self-efficacy scale following the program. This hypothesis could be tested using ANOVA or paired *t* tests to compare the mean self-efficacy scores of participants before and after the program. If the results showed that the mean scores after the program were significantly higher than those from before the program, there would be support for the construct validity of the new self-efficacy scale.

Two primary statistical approaches are used in construct validity assessment. The Pearson product moment correlation is used to test correlational hypotheses. As with criterion validity, there is no standard value of the correlation coefficient that serves as a cut-off score to determine that the criteria for validity have been met. The researcher must rely on what is already known about the relationships among the constructs to make judgments about the adequacy of the validity coefficient as evidence of construct validity. Some of the estimates of expected relationships could be obtained from other studies. To assess group differences using the known-group approach, the *t* test or ANOVA is used. Statistically significant differences are generally needed to support construct validity.

To conduct a construct validity assessment, one begins by formulating one or more hypotheses, ideally based on an explicitly stated theory that includes the construct. Instruments are then selected that measure the other constructs included in the test. Data are gathered from participants who represent the group for which the new instrument is being developed. The hypotheses are tested, and if the relationships are consistent with the hypotheses, evidence is gathered to support the construct validity of the new measure.

If hypotheses are not supported, one possible conclusion is that the new instrument is flawed and does not yield valid scores. However, there are three other possible conclusions that the researcher should consider before deciding that the instrument is not suitable (Cronbach and Meehl, 1955). The theory, which served as the basis for the analysis, may itself be unsound, or the instruments used to measure the other constructs may not meet the minimum standards for reliability and validity. Finally, the methods used to conduct the study may have contributed in some way to measurement error.

Multitrait-Multimethod Matrix

In 1959, Campbell and Fiske described the multitrait-multimethod (MTMM) process for assessing construct validity. In proposing the process, Campbell and Fiske argued that some of the variance shared between traits (constructs) is due to the traits (trait variance) and some is due to the manner in which the traits are measured (method variance). They also maintained that for trait and method variance to be estimated, the assessment of both convergent and discriminant validity is required. Convergent validity is assessed by comparing the same trait as measured by two independent methods. For example, adherence to one's medication schedule might be measured by a self-report diary and by a medication monitoring system called MEMS™ (an electronic surveillance of openings of the cap on a medication bottle) (AARDEX, Ltd., 2005). If the two methods of measuring adherence yield similar results, evidence of convergent validity exists. Discriminant validity is assessed by examining correlations between traits that are dissimilar. In this assessment, correlations between the traits should be low, providing evidence that the traits differ (unlike convergent validity, in which strong positive correlations are desired). A discriminant-validity assessment of a self-report instrument of medication adherence might include the construct of social support. Although there might be a positive correlation between social support and adherence, that correlation is not expected to be particularly strong. If the correlation were strong, the validity of the adherence measure would be questioned.

The MTMM process involves the comparison of two or more traits, each measured by at least two methods. A correlation matrix is used to present the correlations for every possible trait by method comparison. Table 11.5 shows the simplest matrix, with two concepts labeled A and B and two methods labeled 1 and 2. Trait A1 is construct A measured by method 1, and trait A2 is the same construct measured by method 2. Likewise, trait B1 is construct B measured by method 1 and trait B2 is the same construct measured by method 2. Convergent validity for trait A is assessed by comparing A1 with A2 and for trait B by comparing B1 with B2. Discriminant validity for both traits A and B is assessed by comparing A1 with B1, A2 with B2, A1 with B2, and A2 with B1. The matrix is composed of the correlations between these variables, along with the reliability coefficients for each measure. The reliability

TABLE 11.5. EXPECTED PATTERN OF RELATIONSHIPS FOR A MULTITRAIT-MULTIMETHOD MATRIX.

	A1	B1	A2	B2
A1	R[1]			
B1	Low[3]	R		
A2	High[2]	Lowest[4]	R	
B2	Lowest[4]	High[2]	Low[3]	R

coefficients are placed on the diagonal. The matrix is examined for the following expected pattern and strength of correlations:

1. Reliability coefficients, which represent monotrait-monomethod, have the highest values.
2. Correlations between instruments measuring the same trait by different methods (monotrait-heteromethod) should be sufficiently high to provide support for convergent validity.
3. Correlations between instruments measuring different traits using the same method (heterotrait-monomethod) should be lower than the monotrait-heteromethod correlations.
4. Correlations between instruments measuring different traits by different methods (heterotrait-heteromethod) should have the lowest correlations.

To conduct an MTMM validity assessment, the researcher first selects two or more constructs measured by two or more methods. The set of instruments may include a new instrument for which the researcher is gathering evidence to support the validity of the measure. If the researcher is interested only in the validity of a new instrument (A), then only the validity of the new instrument is assessed. Participants are asked to complete all the instruments, and correlations are computed for relationships among the scores on the instruments.

Table 11.6 presents the results of an assessment using two traits, quality of life (QOL) and stigma, and two methods, self-report and interview. Suppose that the focus of this assessment is on the new self-report QOL scale. The results of this assessment show that the reliabilities for the four instruments are good, ranging from .88 to .92. The correlation between QOL as measured by self-report and as measured by interview is .74, which is sufficiently high to provide support for convergent validity. The correlation between QOL and stigma measured by self-report is −.44; measured by interview, it is −.40. Both of these values are moderate, which shows some relationship between the two variables. The relationship is negative, indicating that as

TABLE 11.6. MULTITRAIT-MULTIMETHOD VALIDITY MATRIX FOR QOL AND STIGMA SCALES MEASURED BY SELF-REPORT AND INTERVIEW.

		Self-Report		Interview	
		QOL	Stigma	QOL	Stigma
Self-report	QOL	.92			
	Stigma	−.44	.88		
Interview	QOL	.74	−.22	.90	
	Stigma	−.16	.66	−.40	.92

one's perception of stigma decreases, one's QOL increases. However, these relationships are not as strong as that between the two measures of QOL. The pattern of relationships thus far provides support for discriminant validity, because both of the heterotrait-monomethod correlations are lower than the monotrait-heteromethod correlation. Finally, the correlations between QOL and stigma measured by different methods are evaluated. The correlation between QOL (self-report) and stigma (interview) is −.16 and that between QOL (interview) and stigma (self-report) is −.22. Both correlations are lower than the heterotrait-monomethod correlations providing support for validity. Evaluating the pattern of all the correlations shows that the expected hierarchy of relationships is supported. Thus, in this case, there is support for the validity of the new QOL scale.

The conceptualization underlying the MTMM approach is elegant, yet it is difficult to achieve in practice (Campbell & Russo, 2001). Although many researchers have used MTMM to test the construct validity, few have found the pattern of required correlations, and many have noted validity coefficients (monotrait-heteromethod) lower than other coefficients in the matrix (Fiske & Campbell, 1992). These findings have lead Fiske and Campbell (1992) to caution that MTMM should be used as one method among a set of procedures to assess construct validity and not the sole method.

Validity Issues

When one is assessing validity, it is important to use a large enough sample. Responses from a small number of participants can result in large sampling errors, which reduce statistical power. Under these conditions, the chance of a Type II error increases: that is, the null hypothesis (there is no difference) is accepted when in fact a statistically significant relationship exists. Attenuated correlations due to restriction of range are another possibility (see Chapter Eight). If a test is validated on a group of individuals whose scores do not represent the total range of scores, the validity coefficient can be underestimated. Reliability of instruments should be assessed before validity tests are conducted. Instruments with poor reliability will attenuate or reduce the correlation between variables. To avoid this problem, the researcher should evaluate the reliability of all instruments before the validity assessments.

Summary

In this chapter, we have learned that validity is a unitary concept. There are, however, different approaches to gathering theoretical and empirical evidence to support validity. Although researchers commonly refer to the validity of an instrument, it should be emphasized that *validity* refers to the interpretation and use of the scores and is not a characteristic of the instrument itself. There are several determinants of a person's score on a scale or test. These determinants include characteristics of the instrument itself, characteristics of the person, and characteristics of the setting in which the scale or test is administered. Thus, validity must be assessed among different groups and in different settings. There are varying degrees of validity. Validity is not an all-or-none principle; rather, it is an evolving property. New findings may either enhance validity or detract from validity for a particular group of respondents. Evidence is never complete; thus, the process of validation is continual.

CHAPTER TWELVE

FACTOR ANALYSIS

LEARNING OBJECTIVES

At the end of this chapter, the student should be able to

1. Define the term *factor analysis*.
2. Identify three reasons for using factor analysis in scale development.
3. Describe the steps in the factor analysis process.
4. Apply the factor analysis procedures in the analysis of a scale.
5. Provide a basic interpretation of a factor analysis.

Thus far, we have discussed validity in terms of the way a scale acts when it is subjected to a series of tests. If the scale performs as expected, there is evidence to support the validity of the scale. Another approach to validity assessment is to evaluate the internal structure of the scale. Researchers who develop scales in which items are included that assess two or more dimensions might want to know whether or not the dimensions they have proposed actually exist and whether there are more or fewer dimensions than originally proposed. They might also ask whether there is empirical evidence to support the inclusion of an item within a specific dimension. Scales in which the researcher has not consciously developed items for specific dimensions can also be assessed to determine whether items cluster together to form dimensions or subscales.

In this chapter, we discuss factor analysis (FA), which is a technique used to assess the construct validity of an instrument. FA can also be used to identify weak items and to refine an instrument during early testing. We discuss what FA is and describe its use, both for the refinement of an instrument and for the assessment of construct validity. There are several different FA techniques. Moreover, FA techniques are used to answer a variety of research questions beyond those related to instrument development. However, because of the focus of this book, we will limit our discussion to the use of FA for exploring the internal structure of a scale. Most of this chapter will be devoted to a description of the procedures for conducting an exploratory factor analysis (EFA). Students who want only a brief description of factor analysis may read the first section on exploratory factor analysis, including the definition and conceptual basis, and then skip to the last section, on EFA for factor interpretation. A brief description of confirmatory factor analysis (CFA) concludes the chapter.

Exploratory Factor Analysis

FA is called exploratory factor analysis when it is used early in the development of a scale to identify the number of factors, the correspondence between items and factors, and the quality of items. In this section, we discuss how one uses FA to meet these objectives.

Definition

FA is a technique designed to reduce a set of observed variables (that is, items) to a smaller set of variables that reflects the interrelationships among the observed variables. The new variables are called factors; because they are derived from the data and not directly measured, they are known as unobserved, or latent, variables. Applied specifically to the study of the structure of a scale, the FA process categorizes items (observed or manifest variables) according to the strength of their relationships with other scale items. Items that are more strongly correlated are grouped together and separated from other items, which also cluster together. Each set of related items forms a factor, which is interpreted as a latent (unobserved) variable representing a dimension of the construct measured.

There are three primary reasons for using FA in scale development. The first is to determine whether the number of dimensions originally proposed for a scale exists. Recall that the outcome expectations for healthy eating scale, presented in Chapter Seven, was based on Bandura's model (1997) and developed to measure three dimensions of OE: self-evaluative, social, and physical. Four items were written for each dimension. Using a conventional factor analysis diagram, the proposed internal structure of the scale is presented in Figure 12.1. Each circle represents a latent

FIGURE 12.1. STRUCTURE OF THE OUTCOME EXPECTATIONS FOR HEALTHY EATING SCALE.

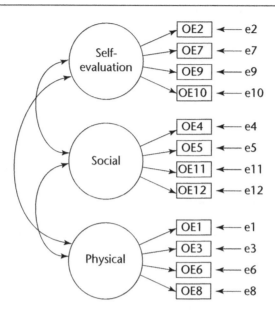

variable corresponding to one dimension; each rectangle, an item. The latent variables are linked to the items by arrows. Thus, we see that item 1 (OE1) was intended to be a measure of the physical dimension of OE (if you eat a healthy diet, you will have more energy), whereas OE4 was written to assess the social dimension (if you eat a healthy diet, your friends will approve). We might expect that respondents who agree that eating a healthy diet will give them more energy (OE1) would also be more likely to agree that eating a healthy diet will help them control their weight (OE6). It would not necessarily follow that people who believe eating a healthy diet will give them more energy would also believe that their friends would approve of their eating a healthy diet. However, we might expect that those who feel their friends would approve (OE4) would also feel that their close relatives would approve (OE12)—from the social dimension. Thus, the expectation is that the items measuring a dimension are more strongly correlated with each other than are items across dimensions. The curved lines connecting the circles imply that the three dimensions are correlated with each other, and the small *e*s represent variance due to measurement error.

The researcher can use FA to determine whether the items written to measure each dimension (that is, self-evaluative, social, and physical) are more strongly correlated with each other than they are with the items written to measure other dimensions of the scale. If there is correspondence, the factor analysis will produce one factor to represent each dimension. In the case of the OE scale, there would be three factors. The items written for each dimension will appear only within the factor that represents that dimension. If the data obtained from a sample of respondents support the proposed scale structure, there is also evidence to support the theoretical framework from which the scale was developed, in this case Bandura's conceptualization of OE.

Sometimes researchers develop items to measure a construct without specifying dimensions during the development process. In this case, the researcher can use FA to determine whether sets of items correlate with each other to form latent variables. In another case, the researcher might have an idea that more than one latent variable exists, but might not be absolutely certain which items belong to which latent variable. For example, the items on the stigma scale presented in Exhibit 12.1 were written to measure the general construct of stigma. It is quite possible that there are underlying latent variables that the researcher did not consider in the original development of the scale. It is possible that the items addressing the person's perception of his or her reaction to having epilepsy (for example, item 7, "I feel embarrassed about my seizure condition") would form one factor and the items addressing the ways in which others react to a person who has seizures (for example, item 1, "People who know that I have a seizure condition treat me differently") would form another factor. Using responses from a sample of participants and FA procedures, the researcher can determine the number and kinds of patterns of relationships that exist among the items.

A third use of FA for instrument development is to identify weak items on a scale. Weak items are those that have low correlations with other scale items and do not appear to adequately represent any latent variable within a scale. Ideally, before conducting an FA, the researcher has written items to measure a construct and has had experts evaluate the items for the scale. Thus, the researcher has some preliminary evidence that the items measure the construct. Despite this evidence, however, there may be items that when put to the test of having respondents answer them will not be correlated as expected with other items. Using the results of FA to identify weak items is similar to using information from an item analysis assessment to identify poor items (Chapter Ten). During the early development of a scale, the researcher is likely to use information from both the item analysis and the FA to make decisions about the retention or deletion of items.

Because factor analysis is based on mathematical and not statistical procedures, it differs from the validity approaches that we have discussed so far. Using statistical analyses for validity assessment, the researcher can state a hypothesis, conduct a statistical test, and use the results of the test to make a decision about accepting or rejecting the hypothesis. Factor analysis yields considerable output but no one number on which to base a decision. The researcher must use both conceptual and quantitative skills to evaluate the output and make decisions about the number of factors,

EXHIBIT 12.1. ITEMS ON THE EPILEPSY STIGMA SCALE.

1. People who know that I have a seizure condition treat me differently.
2. It really doesn't matter what I say to people about my seizure condition, they usually have their minds made up.
3. I always have to prove myself because of the seizure condition.
4. Because of my seizure condition, I have problems developing intimate relationships.
5. In many people's minds, a seizure condition attaches a stigma or label to me.
6. I feel different from other adults because of my seizure condition.
7. I feel embarrassed about my seizure condition.
8. I feel ashamed to tell others about my seizure condition.
9. I feel others are uncomfortable with me because of my seizure condition.
10. I feel others would prefer not to be with me because of my seizure condition.

Source: DiIorio et al., 2003

the items that correspond to each factor, the interpretation of the factors, and the correspondence with the theoretical framework. Fortunately, there are guidelines that can be used to make these decisions, and these are presented below.

Conceptual Basis

Conceptually, the process of factor analyzing a scale is similar to that of placing elements in categories based on similarities. Consider, for example, the following list of physical activities: walking, running, horseback riding, barrel racing, biking, spinning, aerobics, swimming, water aerobics, step class, yoga, karate, isometrics, lawn bowling, weight training, football, rowing, baseball, soccer, tennis, lacrosse, ice skating, table tennis, cricket, horse jumping, golf, water polo, basketball, ice hockey, scuba diving, track, horse racing, kayaking, horse polo, handball, Pilates, squash, racquetball, treadmill, bronco riding, and Stairmaster. A student asked to sort these activities into categories based on their similarities and then to name the categories might produce those listed in Table 12.1. According to the table, the hypothetical student has divided the activities into nine categories. The Team Sports category includes those activities in which teams use a ball to score points. The Aerobic Activities category includes those that promote cardiovascular endurance, and the Horse-Related Activities category includes horses. Notice that the categories are not mutually exclusive. For example, water aerobics, placed under Water Activities, shares some characteristics with aerobic activities. Ice skating and ice hockey share a characteristic—they are performed on the ice—and if they were placed together they could form their own category, Ice

TABLE 12.1. CATEGORIES OF PHYSICAL ACTIVITIES FORMED BY CONCEPTUAL SIMILARITIES.

Aerobic Activities	Bike	Horse-Related	Lawn Activities	Locomotion	Racquet and Net Sports	Strength and Toning	Team Sports	Water Activities
Aerobics	Biking	Barrel racing	Cricket	Ice skating	Handball	Isometrics	Baseball	Rowing
Stairmaster	Spinning	Bronco riding	Golf	Running	Racquetball	Karate	Basketball	Kayaking
Step class		Horseback riding	Lawn bowling	Track	Squash	Pilates	Football	Scuba diving
		Horse racing		Treadmill	Table tennis	Weight training	Handball	Swimming
		Jumping (horse)		Walking	Tennis	Yoga	Ice hockey	Water aerobics
		Polo (horse)			Volleyball		Lacrosse	Water polo
							Soccer	

Sports. Likewise, an argument could be made that weight training and Pilates should be placed in separate categories and that biking and spinning should be added to Aerobic Activities.

FA procedures do much the same thing, that is, sort items by their similarities. One difference, however, is the nature of the process. In the sorting process described earlier, a conceptual approach was used to make decisions about activity placement. FA, on the other hand, uses the responses of participants to items on the scale (that is, empirical data) to place items in categories. The item-item correlation matrix produced to show relationships among individual items is used in the FA. The correlation matrix shows the strength and sign of the relationship of each item with every other item. Items that are strongly related to each other are thought to be similar to each other in some respect, whereas those that have weak correlations are thought to have little in common.

To illustrate an item-item correlation matrix and the other steps in FA, we will use data from a study of HIV risk reduction practices among college students. For this analysis, we include 3,326 respondents who completed a twelve-item condom-use self-efficacy scale (hereafter referred to as the SE scale). Due to space constraints and the fact that it is easier to present some EFA principles with shorter scales, we use eight of the twelve items for some of the examples.

We begin by considering the item-item correlation matrix for eight items from the SE scale. This matrix is presented in Table 12.2. We reordered the items in the matrix to form two groups based on the strength of their correlations. Items within each group (shaded areas) are more strongly correlated with each other than they are with items in the other group (unshaded box). The correlations among items SE1, SE6, SE8, and SE10 range from .494 to .636, and for items SE2, SE4, SE9, and SE11, the correlations range from .602 to .722. Correlations of items across the two groups range from −.038 to .239 (unshaded box). Examining the content of the items (Table 12.2), we see that the first set of items seems to address refusal skills (SE1, SE6, SE8, and SE10) and

TABLE 12.2. CORRELATION MATRIX FOR EIGHT ITEMS ON THE SE SCALE.

	SE1	SE6	SE8	SE10	SE2	SE4	SE9	SE11
SE1	1.0							
SE6	.499	1.0						
SE8	.580	.494	1.0					
SE10	.636	.541	.580	1.0				
SE2	.048	.155	.165	.041	1.0			
SE4	−.021	.083	.101	−.038	.722	1.0		
SE9	.085	.197	.239	.088	.682	.712	1.0	
SE11	.078	.221	.195	.082	.602	.646	.630	1.0

the second set (SE2, SE4, SE9, and SE11) condom-use skills. As we have done here, it is possible to use a visual examination of correlations to determine clusters of items. However, given the complexity of correlation matrices, particularly with a large number of items, more sophisticated procedures are needed to make decisions about grouping items. FA is such a procedure.

How Factor Analysis Works

Factor analysis is a set of mathematical procedures designed to sort items based on their relationships to each other and to identify latent variables that underlie these relationships (Pedhazur & Schmelkin, 1991). The mathematical procedures for factor analysis are elegant but complex. To understand how these procedures work, one should have knowledge of algebra, in particular matrix algebra, and a good grasp of the concepts of variance and latent variables. The student will be pleased to know that we will not discuss mathematical solutions for FA. For those students who are interested in reading more about FA procedures, Comrey and Lee (1992), Kline (1994), and Norman and Streiner (2000) each provide a good introductory background to factor analysis. More advanced texts include Nunnally and Bernstein (1994), Pedhazur and Schmelkin (1991), Pett, Lackey, and Sullivan (2003), and Tabachnick and Fidell (2001). Students who want to explore the mathematical equations themselves should consult Mulaik (1972).

Suffice it to say that factor analysis procedures begin with the item-item correlation matrix and reconfigure the matrix to produce a factor matrix (Tabachnick & Fidell, 2001) (Figure 12.2). In the item-item correlation matrix, each item is correlated with every other item on the scale. The numbers in the main body of the matrix are called correlation coefficients (1), and each gives an indication of the strength and sign of the relationship between two items. In the factor matrix, the items in the scale are correlated with the factors, the new unobserved (latent) variables produced during the factoring process. The numbers in the matrix are called factor loadings (2). Each factor loading gives an indication of the strength and sign of the relationship between an item and the factor. Like correlation coefficients, factor loadings range from –1 to +1 and are interpreted in the same way as correlation coefficients are, with higher values more strongly correlated with the factors.

Steps in Factor Analysis

Figure 12.3 presents the steps in the FA process. These steps guide the following discussion of the SPSS procedures used to conduct FA and the interpretation of the SPSS printout. To illustrate FA, we use the twelve-item SE scale. Though this practical

FIGURE 12.2. RECONFIGURATION OF A CORRELATION MATRIX INTO A FACTOR (STRUCTURE) MATRIX FOR EIGHT ITEMS ON THE SE SCALE.

Correlation Matrix

	SE1	SE6	SE8	SE10	SE2	SE4	SE9	SE11
SE1	1.0							
SE6	.499	1.0						
SE8	.580	.494	1.0					
SE10	.636	.541	.580	1.0				
SE2	.048	.155	.165	.041	1.0			
SE4	−.021	.083	.101	−.038	.722	1.0		
SE9	.085	.197	.239	.088	.682	.712	1.0	
SE11	.078	.494	.195	.082	.602	.646	.630	1.0

1. Correlation coefficient

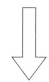

Factor Matrix

2. Factor loading

	Factor	
	1	2
1. Can say no to pressure to have sex	.188	.755
2. Can put condom on without breaking	.806	−.147
4. Can put condom on in dark	.834	−.255
6. Can say no to sex without condom even if really like partner	.299	.596
8. Can say no to sex even if had sex with partner before	.331	.661
9. Can use condom without fumbling	.831	−.085
10. Can say no to sex even if new and attracted to partner	.188	.789
11. Can put condom on even with new partner	.746	−.072

approach does not provide a full appreciation of FA, we hope that the student will gain some understanding of FA for scale development in order to conduct an FA and understand the results of FA presented in published studies.

Basic Requirements for FA

Certain conditions must be met before a set of responses from participants can be analyzed using FA techniques. First, the scale should include items that are measured on a rating scale that consists of at least three response options. For example, a five-point Likert scale that has response choices ranging from *strongly disagree* to *strongly agree* would meet this requirement, whereas a knowledge test with the dichotomous responses of *yes* and *no* would not. Although it is possible to factor analyze scales with dichotomous items, it often requires special techniques to obtain the correlation matrix (Mulaik, 1972). Ideally, responses to each scale item are normally distributed. Tabachnick and Fidell (2001) note that this requirement is often relaxed and that variable transformations can be considered for highly skewed or kurtotic variables. Generally, FA procedures require fairly large sample sizes. Although different authors give different guidelines for the minimal sample size, most agree that small samples (less than 100)

FIGURE 12.3. STEPS IN FACTOR ANALYSIS.

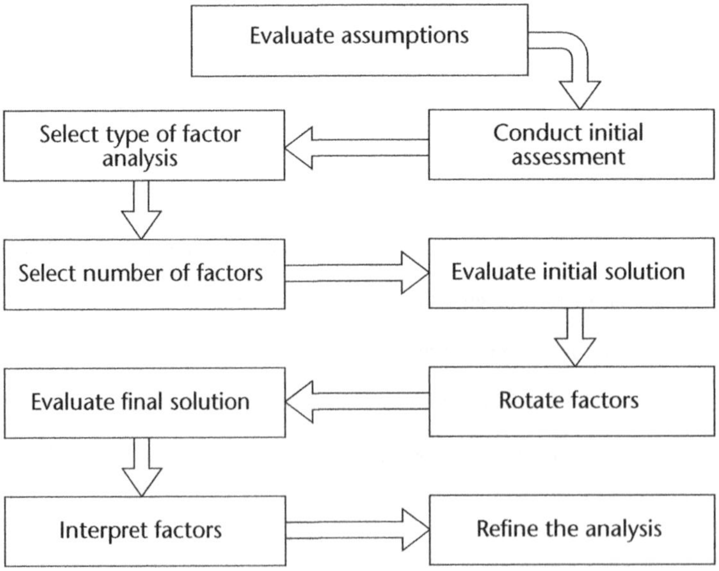

produce unstable results and the larger sample sizes (300 or more) produce more stable factor solutions. Tabachnick and Fidell (2001) recommend at least 300 respondents for factor analysis. Some authors suggest a ratio of participants to items as an estimate of required sample size. Nunnally and Bernstein (1994) recommend including ten participants for every item, whereas Pett, Lackey, and Sullivan (2003) suggest ten to fifteen participants per item.

The first step in FA is to evaluate these basic assumptions. The items on the SE scale are rated on a ten-point response scale using the anchors 1, *not at all sure I can,* to 10, *completely sure I can,* and thus meeting the criterion for the number of response options. The sample size of 3,326 respondents is much greater than that recommended both for respondents per item and for the total sample. To evaluate the distribution of items, we use SPSS to generate a descriptive table that presents the means and standard deviations of the individual items. The SPSS commands at the bottom of the page were used to generate the descriptive table.

Table 12.3 presents the SPSS output for the twelve-item SE scale. The table includes the means, the standard deviations, and the number of respondents for each item. Item means range from 7.60 to 8.88, with standard deviations from 1.866 to 2.743. Although the response-option and sample-size requirements are met, the data show a negative skewing that might be problematic. If necessary, transformations of the data can be considered.

Initial Assessment

The next step is to conduct a preliminary assessment to determine the adequacy of the correlation matrix and the sample size for factor analysis. There are three assessments that can be made to determine the adequacy of the matrix and two for sample adequacy.

To generate a descriptive table:

From the Data Editor Screen:

√Analyze. . . .Data Reduction. . . .√Factor

    Highlight and transfer variables from L→R column

    √Descriptives (Dialog Box)

        √Univariate descriptives

        √Continue

    √OK

TABLE 12.3. SPSS PRINTOUT WITH DESCRIPTIVE STATISTICS FOR THE TWELVE-ITEM SE SCALE.

Descriptive Statistics

		Mean	Std. Deviation	Analysis N
1.	Can say no to pressure to have sex	8.19	2.452	3326
2.	Can put condom on without breaking	7.85	2.601	3326
3.	Can talk to partner about why use condom	8.88	1.866	3326
4.	Can put condom on in dark	7.77	2.743	3326
5.	Can discuss HIV/AIDS prevention w/partner	8.70	1.989	3326
6.	Can say no to sex without condom even if really like partner	8.37	2.407	3326
7.	Can discuss importance of condom use	8.86	1.892	3326
8.	Can say no to sex even if had sex with partner before	8.03	2.551	3326
9.	Can use condom without fumbling	7.60	2.620	3326
10.	Can say no to sex even if new and attracted to partner	8.46	2.453	3326
11.	Can put condom on even with new partner	8.02	2.555	3326
12.	Can convince any sex partner to use condom	8.42	2.232	3326

Evaluation of the Matrix. The tables required to assess both the adequacy of the matrix and the sample are available in the Descriptives dialog box in SPSS (Figure 12.4). The following commands give (1) a correlation matrix and significance tables, (2) a table with Kaiser-Meyer-Olkin (KMO) and Bartlett's test results, and (3) anti-image covariance and correlation matrices.

(The Initial Solution command in the Descriptives dialog box is checked by default. We will review the table from this command in the next section.)

The Coefficients and Significance Levels commands produce a table such as Table 12.4. The upper half of the table is a correlation matrix and the lower half presents the significance levels for the correlations. The first step is to examine the correlation matrix. A visual examination of the item-item correlations within the correlation matrix gives an indication of the strengths of the relationships between items. If all the correlations are near 0, there is not much evidence that the items are related to each other. Thus, it is unlikely that a factor analysis will produce one or more factors that explain correlations among items. A matrix that demonstrates moderate to high correlations among items generally indicates that at least one factor is present. A matrix that demonstrates the possibility of more than one factor consists of items

To conduct a preliminary assessment:

From the Data Editor Screen:

√Analyze. . . .Data Reduction. . . .√Factor

    √Descriptives (dialog box)

        √Coefficients

        √Significance levels

        √Determinant

        √KMO and Bartlett's test of sphericity

        √Anti-image

        √Continue

    √OK

that show moderate to high correlations with some items and low correlations with others. That is, some items "hang together" more than others (Pedhazur & Schmelkin, 1991). This visual examination of a matrix is very difficult when there are more than a few items on the scale, but identifying the existence of relationships among items suggests that the matrix can be factor analyzed.

The correlation matrix for the twelve-item SE scale is presented in the upper half of Table 12.4. The correlations, which range from −.038 to .722, show moderate to high correlations among some items, and low correlations among others. The lower half of the table shows that all but one correlation is statically significant with p values <.001. The p values in this matrix must be evaluated with caution, because the sample size for this data set is very large, so weak correlations (r <.10) are statistically significant. Nonetheless, the pattern of relationships suggests that the data set will be acceptable for factor analysis.

FIGURE 12.4. SPSS DIALOG BOX FOR DESCRIPTIVES COMMAND.

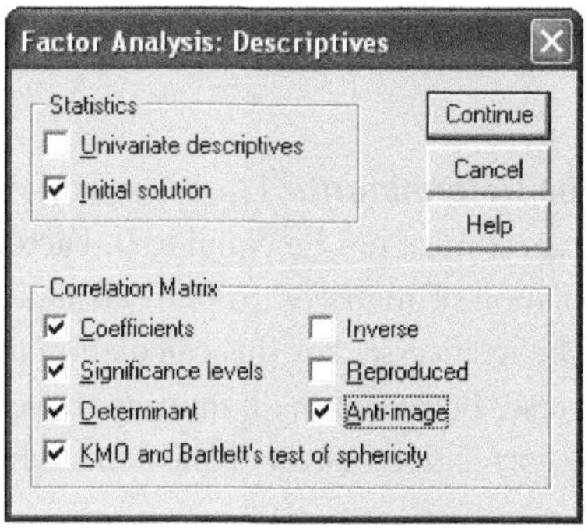

TABLE 12.4. SPSS PRINTOUT OF THE CORRELATION MATRIX FOR THE TWELVE-ITEM SE SCALE.

Correlation Matrix[a]

		Can say no to pressure to have sex	Can put condom on w/o break	Can talk to any partner about why use condom	Can put condom on in dark	Can discuss HIV/AIDS prevention w/ partner	Can say no to sex w/o condom even if really like partner	Can discuss importance of condom use	Can say no to sex w/ partner had sex with before	Can use condom w/o fumbling	Can say no to sex even if new and attracted to person	Can put condom on even w/ new partner	Can convince any sex partner to use condom
Correlation	1. Can say no to pressure to have sex	1.000	.048	.283	−.021	.345	.499	*Moderate to high correlations*			.636	.078	.226
	2. Can put condom on without breaking	.048	1.000	.371	.722	.279	.155				.041	.602	.337
	3. Can talk to any partner about why use condom	.283	.371	1.000	.332	.575	.443	.669	.337	.363	.280	.395	.549
	4. Can put condom on in dark	−.021	.722	.322	1.000	.258	.083	.270	.101	.712	*Low correlations*		.322
	5. Can discuss HIV/AIDS prevention with partner	.345	.279	.575	.258	1.000	.427	.684	.385	.324			.414
	6. Can say no to sex without condom even if really like partner	.499	.155	.443	.083	.427	1.000	.527	.494	.197	.541	.221	.387
	7. Can discuss importance of condom use	.331	.312	.669	.270	.684	.527	1.000	.398	.354	.382	.373	.514
	8. Can say no to sex even if had sex with partner before	.580	.165	.337	.101	.385	.494	.398	1.000	.239	.580	.195	.321
	9. Can use condom without fumbling	.085	.682	.363	.712	.324	.197	.354	.239	1.000	.088	.630	.376
	10. Can say no to sex even if new and attracted to person	.636	.041	.280	−.038	.323	.541	.362	.580	.088	1.000	.082	.249
	11. Can put condom on even with new partner	.078	.602	.395	.646	.321	.221	.373	.195	.630	.082	1.000	.411
	12. Can convince any sex partner to use condom	.226	.337	.549	.322	.414	.387	.514	.321	.376	.249	.411	1.000
Sig. (1-tailed)	1. Can say no to pressure to have sex		.003	.000	.108	.000	.000	.000	.000	.000	.000	.000	.000
	2. Can put condom on without breaking	.003		.000	.000	.000	.000	.000	.000	.000	.009	.000	.000
	3. Can talk to any partner about why use condom	.000	.000		.000	.000	.000	.000	.000	.000	.000	.000	.000
	4. Can put condom on in dark	.108	.000	.000		.000	.000	.000	.000	.000	.015	.000	.000
	5. Can discuss HIV/AIDS prevention with partner	.000	.000	.000	.000		.000	.000	.000	.000	.000	.000	.000
	6. Can say no to sex without condom even if really like partner	.000	.000	.000	.000	.000		.000	.000	.000	.000	.000	.000
	7. Can discuss importance of condom use	.000	.000	.000	.000	.000	.000		.000	.000	.000	.000	.000
	8. Can say no to sex even if had sex with partner before	.000	.000	.000	.000	.000	.000	.000		.000	.000	.000	.000
	9. Can use condom without fumbling	.000	.000	.000	.000	.000	.000	.000	.000		.000	.000	.000
	10. Can say no to sex even if new and attracted to person	.000	.009	.000	.015	.000	.000	.000	.000	.000		.000	.000
	11. Can put condom on even with new partner	.000	.000	.000	.000	.000	.000	.000	.000	.000	.000		.000
	12. Can convince any sex partner to use condom	.000	.000	.000	.000	.000	.000	.000	.000	.000	.000	.000	

a. Determinant = .002

Determinant of the correlation matrix

Evaluation of the Determinant. The second criterion for the matrix is that the determinant of a matrix must not be equal to 0. Factor analysis procedures involve the algebraic manipulation of matrices. In one calculation, the item-item correlation matrix is multiplied by its inverse. For this calculation to be done, the correlation matrix must have an inverse. Because not all matrices have inverses, the first test is to determine whether the correlation matrix of the items submitted for analysis has an inverse.

The determinant of the matrix is a number that provides an indication of whether or not the matrix has an inverse. Though we will not discuss the way in which determinants are calculated, determinants for correlation matrices range in value from 0 to 1. A value of 1 indicates that the correlation matrix is an identity matrix, an indication that factor analysis cannot be done. A value of 0 is also problematic in that a zero indicates that some aspect of the matrix is a linear combination of another aspect, that is, one variable could be the sum of several other variables in the analysis (Pett, Lackey, & Sullivan, 2003). For example, a zero determinant would result from an analysis that included the SAT verbal, the SAT quantitative, and the total SAT score. The total SAT score is a combination of the verbal and the quantitative. A zero determinant could also result if one of the variables has no variation. Although the factor analysis can proceed under these circumstances, SPSS is likely to generate an error message stating that the matrix is not positive definite, meaning that it does not have an inverse and therefore should not be factored (Pett, Lackey, and Sullivan, 2003). Eliminating the redundant (SAT total) variable or variables with little to no variation should solve the problem. A determinant value between 0 and 1 is desirable and indicates that the correlation matrix has an inverse, and thus that factor analysis procedures are possible.

The Determinants command gives a value listed at the bottom left of the correlation matrix table (Table 12.4). The determinant of the SE scale matrix is .002, which is within the acceptable range.

Test for an Identity Matrix. The third test is to examine the matrix to determine whether or not it is an identity matrix. An identity matrix is one in which the numbers on the diagonal are equal to 1, and the numbers off the diagonal are equal to 0. The traditional item-item correlation matrix has 1's on the diagonal, representing the correlation of an item with itself. Most matrices produced to show correlations between items will not have all zeroes in the off-diagonal spaces. However, if items in a set have very little in common with each other, the correlations might be low and in fact close to 0. In this case, the matrix might be close to an identity matrix and it might not be possible to factor it.

To determine whether the matrix is an identity matrix, the researcher can first visually examine the correlation matrix looking for low or near-zero values. Mulaik (2005) notes that if several correlations are greater than $\frac{2}{\sqrt{N-3}}$, the matrix is unlikely to be an identity matrix. In addition, the researcher can conduct Bartlett's test of sphericity. This statistical test compares the correlation matrix of the selected items with an identity matrix. The null hypothesis is that the correlation matrix is an identity matrix, and the alternative hypothesis is that it is not an identity matrix. Thus, for factor analysis to be conducted, the null hypothesis should be rejected. When the null hypothesis is rejected, the values of Bartlett's test (a chi-square statistic) will be large and significant, with a p value of less than .05. When the sample size is large, Bartlett's test may be significant even if the correlation matrix is an identity matrix (Tabachnick & Fidell, 2001). Thus, it is also important to visually examine the correlation matrix to make sure that at least moderate correlations exist among some variables.

The commands for the KMO and Bartlett's test of sphericity give the output for both tests in one table (Table 12.5). The Bartlett's chi-square value for the SE scale is 20,780.313 and is statistically significant. Because of the large sample size, the correlation matrix is also examined visually to make certain that it is not an identity matrix. The evaluation we conducted earlier shows that there are moderate to high correlations among groups of items, indicating that the matrix is not an identity matrix.

Tests of Sampling Adequacy

There are two tests available to assess sampling adequacy. The first is the KMO for sample adequacy. This test compares the differences of two matrices: the item-item correlation matrix and a second matrix of partial correlations among the items. Partial correlations are those correlations between items in which the effects of other items are taken out. When items are moderately or highly correlated with each other, the correlation between any two items with the effect of the other items that are taken out (partial correlation) will be small. Thus, the partial correlation matrix will consist of relatively low correlations in the case in which a set of items shows moderate to high correlations in the original item-item correlation matrix. KMO values range from 0 to 1; those closer to 1 correspond to an item-item correlation matrix with stronger relationships among items. Pett, Lackey, and Sullivan (2003) suggest that the KMO value be above .70. The KMO value for the SE scale is .886, which meets this criterion (Table 12.5).

The second test to assess sampling adequacy is called the Measure of Sampling Adequacy (MSA) test. The KMO gives a value to assess the sampling adequacy for the entire matrix, whereas an MSA is calculated for each item. As with the KMO, the

TABLE 12.5. SPSS PRINTOUT OF THE KMO AND BARTLETT'S TEST OF SPHERICITY FOR THE TWELVE-ITEM SE SCALE.

KMO and Bartlett's Test

Kaiser-Meyer-Olkin Measure of Sampling Adequacy		.886	>.70: meets criterion
Bartlett's Test of Sphericity	Approx. Chi-Square	20780.313	
	df	66	Significant: meets criterion
	Sig.	.000	

calculation of MSAs uses correlations and partial correlations for items and provides an indication of the strength of the relationship between an item and the other items in the matrix (Pett, Lackey, and Sullivan, 2003). The values of MSAs range from 0 to 1; values closer to 1 reflect more interrelationships. The MSA for each item should be above .70 (Pett, Lackey, and Sullivan, 2003).

The Anti-image command in SPSS gives a matrix with the MSAs on the diagonal and partial correlations on the off-diagonals. The Anti-image command provides both the covariance and the correlation matrix. It is best to skip the unstandardized covariance matrix and evaluate the correlation matrix. Table 12.6 presents the anti-image correlation matrix for the SE scale. The MSAs are located on the diagonal and range from .836 to .937. All meet the criterion of .70, indicating adequate sampling. If some of the items do not meet the criterion, Pett, Lackey, and Sullivan (2003) suggest removing these items and refactoring the matrix. If the items are included, an error message might appear, stating "Not positive definite or ill conditioned matrix"; this suggests that it is unwise to continue with factor analysis procedures.

Selection of the Type of Factor Analysis

After the correlation matrix has been evaluated and the researcher feels confident that the matrix is factorable and that the sample size is adequate, the next step is to select the type of FA procedure. There are two major types: principal components analysis (PCA) and common factor analysis (common FA). There are conceptual and analytical differences between these two approaches (Mulaik, 1987, 1990).

PCA is a data reduction method in which a large set of observed variables (items) is reduced to a smaller set of factors (called components in PCA). In the algebraic computations, PCA uses the typical item-item correlation matrix with 1's on the diagonal and includes the total variance available among the variables in the computation of factors. According to Pedhazur and Schmelkin (1991), the aim of PCA is to extract the most variance from a set of items to produce a smaller set of components (factors). The resulting components are weighted sums of observed variables (items) and are completely observed. Components can be thought of as dependent variables and the scale items as independent variables (Pedhazur & Schmelkin, 1991). Moreover, components are primarily descriptive variables applicable only to the correlation (covariance) matrix from which they were produced.

The primary purpose of common FA, on the other hand, is to identify latent constructs among a set of observed variables. These factors are latent variables that are not observed and unlike components, common factors can have the same relationship to observed variables from one covariance matrix to the next (Mulaik, 2004). For common factor analysis, the correlation matrix used in the computations replaces the 1's on the diagonal with communality estimates (these will be explained later). The goal

TABLE 12.6. SPSS PRINTOUT OF THE ANTI-IMAGE CORRELATION MATRIX FOR THE TWELVE-ITEM SE SCALE.

Anti-Image Matrices

Anti-Image Correlation	1. Can say no to pressure to have sex	.843[a]	.002	-.031	.026	-.096	-.148	.039	-.284	.023	-.372	.020	.021
	2. Can put condom on without breaking	.002	.880[a]	-.090	-.386	.013	-.003	-.002	-.012	-.269	.006	-.139	-.002
	3. Can talk to partner about why use condom	-.031	-.090	.906[a]	-.047	-.171	-.083	-.324	.003	.037	.017	-.035	-.249
	4. Can put condom on in dark	.026	-.386	-.047	.836[a]	-.033	.065	.032	.035	-.351	.064	-.263	-.018
	5. Can discuss HIV/AIDS prevention with partner	-.096	.013	-.171	-.033	.893[a]	-.008	-.424	-.067	-.038	.005	-.007	.002
	6. Can say no to sex without condom even if really like partner	-.148	-.003	-.083	.065	-.008	.921[a]	-.197	-.107	-.008	-.227	-.050	-.090
	7. Can discuss importance of condom use	.039	-.002	-.324	.032	-.424	-.197	.867[a]	-.022	-.044	-.054	-.055	-.126
	8. Can say no to sex even if had sex with partner before	-.284	-.012	.003	.035	-.067	-.107	-.022	.895[a]	-.112	-.264	-.007	-.065
	9. Can use condom without fumbling	.023	-.269	.037	-.351	-.038	-.008	-.044	-.112	.886[a]	.000	-.199	-.058
	10. Can say no to sex even if new and attracted to partner	-.372	.006	.017	.064	.005	-.227	-.054	-.264	.000	.842[a]	.011	-.014
	11. Can put condom on even with new partner	.020	-.139	-.035	-.263	-.007	-.050	-.055	-.007	-.199	.011	.924[a]	-.125
	12. Can convince any sex partner to use condom	.021	-.002	-.249	-.018	.002	-.090	-.126	-.065	-.058	-.014	-.125	.937[a]

MSA values

a. Measures of Sampling Adequacy (MSA)

of common FA is to explain shared or common variance among the items, and thus variance unique to each item is not considered in the computation of the factors as it is in PCA. Because the results of PCA and common FA of the same data often look very similar, especially when the factor loadings are high, some believe that either method can be used. Thus, PCA is frequently selected for scale assessment. Although controversy abounds, most theorists prefer common factor analysis for developing theory (Mulaik, 1990; Preacher & MacCallum, 2003). In the discussion here, we use maximum likelihood analysis, a type of common factor analysis, to demonstrate the factor analysis procedures. Other types of common factor analysis include principal axis factoring, unweighted least squares, and generalized least squares.

Initial Extraction. To begin the actual FA process, select the SPSS commands for the initial solution that follows. For this example, we use the default command for selecting number of factors (found under the Extraction command Figure 12.5). Strategies for selecting the number of factors will be explained shortly.

The output from these commands consists of an initial solution table (Table 12.7), a factor matrix (Table 12.8), a communalities table (Table 12.9), a scree plot (Figure 12.6), and a goodness of fit test (Table 12.10). Each is explained below.

The results of the initial extraction provide an opportunity to define some terms associated with factor analysis. The first two terms are *eigenvalues* and *communalities.* Recall that FA reconfigures the variance within a correlation matrix (Figure 12.2). This new configuration of variance can be examined in two ways. One way is the amount of variance explained by each factor (eigenvalue), and the other is the percentage of variance in each item explained by all the factors (communality).

To understand how these variances are computed, it is important to know that the total amount of variance in a set of items is equal to the number of items. Recall that the variance of a standardized variable (the correlation of an item with itself in a correlation matrix) is 1.0. These 1's are found on the diagonal of an item-item correlation

FIGURE 12.5. SPSS DIALOG BOX FOR EXTRACTION COMMANDS.

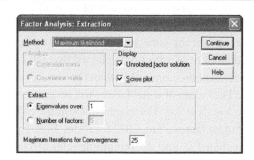

To begin the factor analysis procedure:

From the Data Editor Screen:

√Analyze. . . .Data Reduction. . . .√Factor

    √Descriptives (dialog box)

        √Initial Solution (default)

        √Continue (this will close dialog box)

    √Extraction (dialog box)

        √Maximum likelihood (from pull down menu)

        √Unrotated factor solution (default)

        √Scree plot

        √Eigenvalue >1 (default)

        √Continue

    √OK

matrix. The total amount of variance for a twelve-item scale is the sum of the variances for all the items. Because the variance for each item is 1, and there are twelve items, the total variance is 12. As we mentioned earlier, PCA uses all of the variance to extract the components, whereas common FA uses only shared variance to extract factors. This process of using the variance to extract components or factors is commonly referred to as the *extraction of factors from a matrix*. In both PCA and common FA, the first component (factor) extracts the most variance possible from the matrix, leaving some unexplained variance. The second component (factor) then extracts the most variance possible from the remaining variance, also leaving some unexplained variance. The third component (factor) extracts the most variance possible from the remainder, and the process continues until there is no more variance to extract (Pedhazur & Schmelkin, 1991).

Eigenvalues. In the SPSS printout, the initial extraction always shows that the total number of factors is equal to the number of items (Table 12.7). Thus, for the twelve-item scale, there are twelve factors on the initial extraction printout (1). (Remember that the factors are not the same as the items, even though they are the same in number.) The total amount of variance explained by each factor is called an eigenvalue. Each factor may explain more or less than the amount of variance in a standardized variable (1.0). The values of some factors will be greater than 1.0 and those of other factors will be less than 1.0. The eigenvalues on the SPSS printout for the SE scale range from .253 for factor 12 to 4.977 for factor 1 (2). Factors 1, 2, and 3 have eigenvalues greater than 1.0, and the remaining ones are less than 1.0 (or less than the amount of variance explained by a single item). The factors with eigenvalues greater than 1.0 will form the main factors when the default option for selecting factors in SPSS is used (3).

The third column in Table 12.7 gives the percentage of the total variance explained by each factor (4). The percentage of variance explained by each factor is obtained by dividing the value of the eigenvalue for each factor by the total variance, which is equal to the number of factors. The first component of the SE scale has a value of 4.977 and total variance is 12. The percentage of variance explained by component 1 is computed as follows:

$$\frac{4.977}{12} = .4147 \times 100 = 41.47\%.$$

Factor 1 explains 41.47 percent of the variance in this set of items (4). The second factor accounts for 20.5 percent and the third for 8.7 percent. The fourth column of Table 12.7 shows the cumulative percentage that is calculated by adding each successive percentage (5). Although the goal of FA is to extract fewer factors than items, the initial solution gives information about all the factors. A second solution, called the extracted solution, gives only information about the factors selected for extraction (6). The extraction sums of squared loadings give the amount of variance explained by the factors.

The values of the eigenvalues of the extracted factors can be computed using the factor matrix (Table 12.8). The values on the factor matrix are referred to as factor loadings. The eigenvalue for each factor is found by squaring each factor loading and summing the scores (1).

Thus, the eigenvalue for Factor 1 in Table 12.8 is:

$$.403^2 + .661^2 + .707^2 + .646^2 + .663^2 + .546^2 + .752^2 +$$
$$.511^2 + .700^2 + .412^2 + .665^2 + .613^2 = 4.560.$$

The value obtained is 4.560, which is the same as that in the Extraction Sums of Squared Loadings (6) shown in Table 12.7.

Communality. Communality is the percentage of variance in each item explained by all factors. The communalities of the items for the SE scale are presented in Table 12.9. The column labeled Initial presents the communalities of items based on all factors. The column labeled Extraction presents the communalities based on the extracted factors. The communalities for the extracted factors can be computed using the factor matrix (Table 12.8). The communality for each item is found by summing the row of squared factor loadings (2).

TABLE 12.7. SPSS PRINTOUT OF THE INITIAL SOLUTION FOR THE TWELVE-ITEM SE SCALE.

> 2. Amount of variance explained by a factor

> 1. Always as many factors as there are items

> 4. Percentage of variance explained by a factor

> 6. Factors selected for extraction; sum of squared factor loadings on the factor matrix

Total Variance Explained

Factor	Initial Eigenvalues			Extraction Sums of Squared Loadings			Rotation
	Total	% of Variance	Cumulative %	Total	% of Variance	Cumulative %	Total
1	4.977	41.477	41.477	4.560	37.996	37.996	3.901
2	2.467	20.557	62.034	2.141	17.838	55.834	3.012
3	1.054	8.786	70.819	.709	5.907	61.741	3.406
4	.609	5.079	75.898				
5	.498	4.154	80.052				
6	.422	3.518	83.750				
7	.407	3.395	86.965				
8	.375	3.122	90.087				
9	.360	2.998	93.085				
10	.302	2.519	95.605				
11	.275	2.289	97.894				
12	.253	2.106	100.000				

Extraction method: maximum likelihood

> 3. Eigenvalues greater than 1.0 will be main factors

> 5. Cumulative percentage

The communality for SE10 in Table 12.8 is calculated

$$.412^2 + .599^2 + .354^2 = .655.$$

Note on Table 12.9 that the value of the communality for SE10 after extraction is .655.

Because the number of extracted factors is less than the total number of factors, the percentage of variance explained for the extracted factors does not include their shared variance with the factors that are not included in the final solution. Thus, the communality for each item will be different from that obtained for the initial extraction.

Communalities provide an idea of which items are best represented in the factor solution. Those with high communalities have more variance in common with the selected factors, whereas those with low values are not well represented.

TABLE 12.8. SPSS PRINTOUT FOR THE UNROTATED FACTOR MATRIX FOR THE TWELVE-ITEM SE SCALE.

Factor Matrix[a]

	Factor		
	1	2	3
1. Can say no to pressure to have sex	.403	.572	.358
2. Can put condom on without breaking	.661	−.470	.132
3. Can talk to partner about why use condom	.707	.157	−.281
4. Can put condom on in dark	.646	−.583	.122
5. Can discuss HIV/AIDS prevention with partner	.663	.254	−.255
6. Can say no to sex without condom even if really like partner	.546	.462	6.700E−02
7. Can discuss importance of condom use	.752	.292	−.363
8. Can say no to sex even if had sex with partner before	.511	.444	.311
9. Can use condom without fumbling	.700	−.420	.154
10. Can say no to sex even if new and attracted to person	.412	.599	.354
11. Can put condom on even with new partner	.665	−.356	5.700E−02
12. Can convince any sex partner to use condom	.613	7.852E−02	−.135

1. Eigenvalue for Factor 1: square each number and sum

2. Communality for Item 10: square each number and sum

Extraction method: maximum likelihood.
[a]Three factors extracted. Four iterations required.

TABLE 12.9. SPSS PRINTOUT OF THE COMMUNALITIES TABLE FOR THE TWELVE-ITEM SE SCALE.

Communalities

	Initial	Extraction
1. Can say no to pressure to have sex	.495	.618
2. Can put condom on without breaking	.596	.676
3. Can talk to partner about why use condom	.543	.603
4. Can put condom on in dark	.652	.772
5. Can discuss HIV/AIDS prevention with partner	.513	.569
6. Can say no to sex without condom even if really like partner	.466	.515
7. Can discuss importance of condom use	.626	.782
8. Can say no to sex even if had sex with partner before	.469	.556
9. Can use condom without fumbling	.612	.690
10. Can say no to sex even if new and attracted to partner	.516	.655
11. Can put condom on even with new partner	.523	.573
12. Can convince any sex partner to use condom	.392	.400

1. Communalities before extraction

2. Communalities after extraction

Extraction method: maximum likelihood.

Number of Factors. The goal of factor analysis is to extract a smaller number of factors that explain the variation among the larger set of items. Only those factors that explain an appreciable amount of variance in the data are retained. The default in SPSS is to extract only those factors with initial eigenvalues greater than 1.0. In Table 12.7, you see in column 2 (3) that there are three factors with eigenvalues greater than 1.0, ranging from 1.054 to 4.977. The total percentage of variance explained by these three components is 70.8 percent.

This criterion, called the Kaiser-Guttman rule, is the most widely used method in scale development for selecting the number of factors to retain (Guttman, 1954; Kaiser, 1960). This rule is based on the fact that the variance extracted by any one factor should be greater than the variance for any one item, which is 1.0. Although it is the default in SPSS, it is generally recognized that the Kaiser-Guttman rule can overestimate or underestimate the number of factors to retain (Mulaik, 2004; Pett, Lackey, and Sullivan, 2003).

A second procedure to determine the number of factors to extract is the scree plot. Cattell (1966) proposed graphing the eigenvalues to visually display the relationship among the factors. Figure 12.6 shows the scree plot for the SE scale. The graph shows the higher eigenvalues on the left sloping down and then tapering off, with the lower values on the right. Cattell (1966) named the plot after scree, which consists of the small stones that pile up at the bottom of a mountain. When the height of a mountain is measured, the scree, or rubble, at the bottom is ignored (Nunnally & Bernstein, 1994). Applying this analogy to factor extraction suggests that the researcher retain only those factors on the vertical slope and ignore the ones that form the scree. In other words, the researcher should retain those factors above the point at which the line changes to a gradual descent (Preacher & MacCallum, 2003). The scree plot in Figure 12.6 shows a clear separation between factors 3 and 4, where the scree appears to begin. This suggests a three-factor solution.

When conducting a maximum likelihood common FA, as we have done with the SE scale, one can also examine the goodness-of-fit test (Table 12.10). If a sufficient number of factors has been extracted, the chi-square statistic will be nonsignificant. You will note in Table 12.10 that the chi-square statistic for a three-factor solution is statistically significant for the SE scale. In order to make sure there were no more meaningful factors to exact, we ran the analysis again requesting a four-factor, a five-factor, and a six-factor solution. The chi-square values for both the four- and five-factor solutions were statistically significant. Though the chi-square value for the six-factor solution was not significant, suggesting the ideal number of factors, the meaning of three of the six factors was not as clear as that of the three-factor solution. Likewise, the three-factor solution provided a better interpretation of the meaning of the factors than did the four- and five-factor solutions. Thus the three-factor solution was retained as the

FIGURE 12.6. SPSS PRINTOUT OF THE SCREE PLOT FOR THE TWELVE-ITEM SE SCALE.

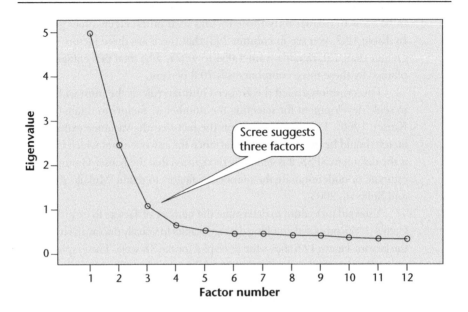

TABLE 12.10. SPSS PRINTOUT OF GOODNESS-OF-FIT TEST FOR THE TWELVE-ITEM SE SCALE.

Goodness-of-Fit Test

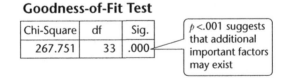

Chi-Square	df	Sig.
267.751	33	.000

$p < .001$ suggests that additional important factors may exist

ideal for this analysis. It should be noted that the chi-square statistic is sensitive to large samples and thus it was not surprising to obtain a significant chi-square for our sample of over 3,000 respondents.

Researchers should consider all available criteria including interpretability to select the number of factors to retain rather than relying solely on the Kaiser-Guttman criterion. To request a specific number of factors in SPSS, open the Extraction dialog box and select "number of factors" at the bottom. Then enter the desired number.

Rotation of Factors

The next step in the factor analysis process is to rotate the factors. Factors are generally rotated to make it easier to interpret their underlying meanings. The interpretation of a factor involves the selection of items that have high factor loadings on it. The content of these items is examined for similarities, and the factor is *named*, or interpreted, based on these similarities. Thus, factors are easier to interpret when (1) each factor has some items with high loadings and some with low loadings and (2) each item has a high loading on one factor and low loadings on the remaining factors (Pedhazur & Schmelkin, 1991). Unrotated factor matrices usually do not display this simple structure, making interpretation difficult.

The factor matrix of the SE scale (Table 12.8) is an unrotated matrix. You can see that there are similar factor loadings for some items on two or more factors. For example, SE10 has a factor loading of .412 on factor 1 and .599 on factor 2. The similar loadings make it difficult to "assign" SE10 to one of the two factors. When items have similar loadings on factors, the situation is referred to as factor complexity or *cross-loading* of items. As we will see later, if the factor matrix is rotated, items will load more strongly on one factor and more weakly on the others.

Factor rotation can be displayed in geometric space by the use of graphs. On such a graph, each factor is represented by a line, and each item is represented by a point. The number of factors determines the number of dimensions in space. A three-factor matrix requires three dimensions, a four-factor matrix requires four dimensions, and so forth. Because it is easier to present an example of factor rotation in two-dimensional space, a FA analysis was conducted using only eight items from the SE scale. These items represent two of the three factors listed in Table 12.8. An item-item correlation matrix for these eight items was presented in Table 12.2. The unrotated factor matrix for these eight items is displayed in Table 12.11. Here we see that there are two columns, representing the two factors, and eight rows, one for each item. Each item has a factor loading on each factor. The values range from .188 to .834 on factor 1 and −.255 to .789 on factor 2.

The information in Table 12.11 can be represented on a graph such as the one in Figure 12.7. On the graph, the *x*-axis is denoted as factor 1, and the *y*-axis as factor 2. The *x*-axis and *y*-axis have values ranging from −1 to +1 and intersect each other at the origin (0,0). Each item from the factor matrix can be plotted on the graph using the factor loadings on the two factors. The factor loadings can be considered coordinates (that is, *x* and *y*) and plotted on the graph with the *x*-axis representing one factor (factor 1) and the *y*-axis representing the other (factor 2). For example, the point (.831, −.085) represents item SE9 and the point (.299, .596) represents item SE6.

Notice on the graph that the items form two clusters. These clusters are not readily apparent from the values of the factor loadings on the unrotated factor matrix

TABLE 12.11. SPSS PRINTOUT OF THE UNROTATED FACTOR MATRIX FOR EIGHT ITEMS ON THE SE SCALE.

Factor Matrix[a]

	Factor	
	1	**2**
1. Can say no to pressure to have sex	.188	.755
2. Can put condom on without breaking	.806	−.147
4. Can put condom on in dark	.834	−.255
6. Can say no to sex without condom even if really like partner	.299	.596
8. Can say no to sex even if had sex with partner before	.331	.661
9. Can use condom without fumbling	.831	−.085
10. Can say no to sex even if new and attracted to partner	.188	.789
11. Can put condom on even with new partner	.746	−.072

(Table 12.11). On the graph, however, the clusters suggest that some of the items "hang together." Rotating the lines around their axes (like rotating the hands of a clock), so that the *y*-axis intersects one cluster of items and the *x*-axis intersects the other, will yield new coordinate values (factor loadings) that are more consistent with simple structure. Simple structure exists when the items that fit with factor 1 fall near or on the *x*-axis and the items for factor 2 fall near or on the *y*-axis.

The goal of factor rotation is to rotate the *x*-axis and the *y*-axis so that the lines are as close as possible to the clusters of items. When the *x*-axis and the *y*-axis are rotated, the values of the coordinates that define each point (item) on the new line change. The items closer to the *x*-axis have higher values for the *x* coordinate and lower values for the *y* coordinate, and vice versa. The changes in values are reflected in the new matrix (the rotated factor matrix), in which the factor loading values are consistent with the *x* and *y* coordinates following rotation.

The rotated factor matrix for the eight items of the SE scale is presented in Table 12.12. These values are plotted in Figure 12.8. Notice that each factor has some items with high values and some with low values. Notice also that each item has a high value on one factor and a low value on the other. When plotted, the items fall closer to either the *x*-axis or the *y*-axis, indicating a higher value on one axis and a lower value on the other. With this type of pattern, it is easier to identify the items that define a factor.

The type of rotation presented with the SE scale is called oblique rotation. In oblique rotation, the *x*-axis and *y*-axis lines are moved independently of each other to obtain the best-fitting line. Oblique rotation is used when the researcher believes that the factors are related to each other. Another type of rotation is called orthogonal

FIGURE 12.7. SCATTERPLOT OF FACTOR LOADINGS FOR THE UNROTATED FACTOR MATRIX FOR THE EIGHT-ITEM SE SCALE.

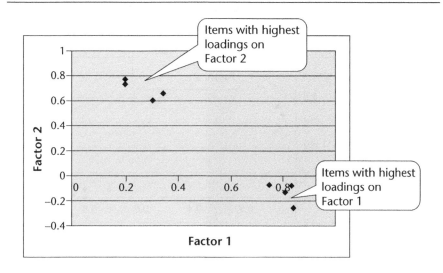

TABLE 12.12. SPSS PRINTOUT OF THE ROTATED FACTOR (PATTERN) MATRIX FOR EIGHT ITEMS ON THE SE SCALE.

Pattern Matrix

		Factor	
		1	2
1.	Can say no to pressure to have sex	−.076	.787
2.	Can put condom on without breaking	.820	−.005
4.	Can put condom on in dark	.883	−.107
6.	Can say no to sex without condom even if really like partner	.083	.648
8.	Can say no to sex even if had sex with partner before	.091	.719
9.	Can use condom without fumbling	.823	.061
10.	Can say no to sex even if new and attracted to partner	−.088	.821
11.	Can put condom on even with new partner	.737	−.060

Extraction method: maximum likelihood.

Rotation method: oblimin with Kaiser normalization.

[a] Rotation converged in three iterations.

FIGURE 12.8. SCATTERPLOT OF FACTOR LOADINGS FOR THE ROTATED FACTOR (PATTERN) MATRIX FOR THE EIGHT-ITEM SE SCALE.

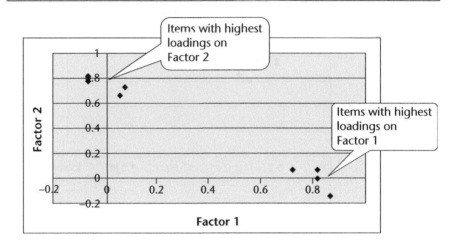

rotation. In orthogonal rotation, the 90-degree angle between the x-axis and the y-axis is maintained throughout the rotation. This type of rotation is used when the researcher believes that the factors are not correlated.

The SPSS dialog box for the selection of the type of rotation is presented in Figure 12.9. There are two types of oblique rotation: direct oblimin and promax. Direct oblimin was selected for the SE scale. Several forms of orthogonal rotation are available in SPSS: varimax, quartimax, and equamax. Selecting the Loading Plots command gives a graph of the items on the rotated factors.

These commands give the output presented in Tables 12.13 and 12.14 and the scatterplot in Figure 12.10. Common FA generates two rotated factor matrices and a correlation matrix. The factor loadings in the structure matrix are equivalent to zero order correlations between the items and factors (Pett, Lackey, and Sullivan, 2003). The factor loadings of the pattern matrix are partial beta weights and are like regression coefficients, indicating how much a unit change of a latent variable produces a change in the observed variable. Notice that the matrices meet the criteria for simple structure because each item loads highly on only one factor and each factor has a mixture of items that have high and low loadings. Either the structure matrix or the pattern matrix is used to interpret the factors. Authors differ on their preference. For example, Pett, Lackey, and Sullivan (2003) support the use of the structure matrix, whereas Mulaik (2004) and Tabachnick and Fidell (2001) prefer the pattern matrix.

FIGURE 12.9. SPSS DIALOG BOX FOR ROTATION COMMANDS.

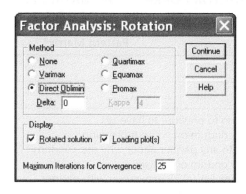

To rotate factors:

From the Data Editor Screen:

√Analyze. . . . .Data Reduction. . . .√Factor

 √Rotation (dialog box)

  √Direct oblimin

  √Rotated solution (default)

  √Loading plots

  √Continue

 √OK

  Table 12.14 presents the correlations among the factors. Notice that factors 1 and 2 are more highly correlated than are factors 2 and 3. Figure 12.10 shows the scatterplot generated from the Loading Plots command. Note the three clusters of items.

  There are a few points to remember about factor rotation. Only the extracted factors (not all the initial factors) are rotated. However, if there is only one factor in the unrotated matrix, there is no need for rotation and no rotated matrix is printed. Rotating the matrix changes the values of the factor loadings, but rotation does not change the total amount of variance explained by the factors.

Interpretation of Factors

  After all this work, we are finally ready to interpret the factors. Remember that in common FA, factors are considered latent variables. The goal of common FA is to identify the hypothetical variable that underlies a set of items that load on a factor (Mulaik, 2003).

TABLE 12.13. SPSS PRINTOUT OF THE ROTATED FACTOR MATRICES AND FACTOR CORRELATION MATRIX FOR THE TWELVE-ITEM SE SCALE.

Pattern Matrix[a]

	Factor		
	1	2	3
1. Can say no to pressure to have sex	−.043	.811	−.025
2. Can put condom on without breaking	−.011	.011	.826
3. Can talk to any partner about why use condom	.756	−.031	.071
4. Can put condom on in dark	−.047	−.072	.904
5. Can discuss HIV/AIDS prevention with partner	.737	.044	−.017
6. Can say no to sex without condom even if really like partner	.352	.475	−.044
7. Can discuss importance of condom use	.929	−.024	−.069
8. Can say no to sex even if had sex with partner before	.022	.711	.109
9. Can use condom without fumbling	−.001	.072	.820
10. Can say no to sex even if new and attracted to partner	−.024	.826	−.044
11. Can put condom on even with new partner	.126	.002	.686
12. Can convince any sex partner to use condom	.498	.052	.179

Structure Matrix

	Factor		
	1	2	3
1. Can say no to pressure to have sex	.390	.784	.050
2. Can put condom on without breaking	.399	.102	.822
3. Can talk to any partner about why use condom	.774	.392	.437
4. Can put condom on in dark	.356	.009	.873
5. Can discuss HIV/AIDS prevention with partner	.753	.447	.350
6. Can say no to sex without condom even if really like partner	.591	.663	.185
7. Can discuss importance of condom use	.882	.478	.384
8. Can say no to sex even if had sex with partner before	.466	.736	.204
9. Can use condom without fumbling	.440	.168	.828
10. Can say no to sex even if new and attracted to partner	.408	.807	.041
11. Can put condom on even with new partner	.464	.152	.748
12. Can convince any sex partner to use condom	.614	.346	.429

TABLE 12.14. FACTOR CORRELATION MATRIX.

Factor	1	2	3
1	1.000	.549	.490
2	.549	1.000	.118
3	.490	.118	1.000

Rotation method: oblimin with Kaiser normalization.

[a] Rotation converged in seven iterations.

FIGURE 12.10. SPSS-GENERATED SCATTERPLOT OF ROTATED FACTOR MATRIX FOR THE TWELVE-ITEM SE SCALE.

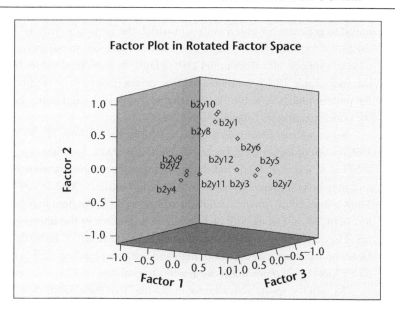

For each factor, items that have large loadings are isolated. The content of this selected group of items is examined. This is a conceptual process in which the researcher carefully evaluates items to identify similarities. Generally, the two or three items with the highest loadings on a factor are evaluated first to determine common defining characteristics. Then the other items in the set are evaluated to ascertain whether they have the same defining characteristics as the items with the highest loadings. The factor is interpreted or "named" according to that which is common to items with the highest loadings, but absent in items that have low or near zero loadings (Mulaik, 2004).

Recall the list of sports activities presented at the beginning of this chapter. A student was given the task of classifying these activities according to common characteristics and then naming the categories. The process of naming groups of items that *load* on a factor is similar to the student's task of labeling the categories of sports activities. The student used the characteristics that the sports had in common to label each group of activities. In Table 12.13, we see that there are four items that load strongly on factor 1: SE3, SE5, SE7, and SE12, and the factor loadings range from .498 to .929. The factor loadings on the other items are low, with most close to zero. These latter items do not contribute much to the interpretation of the factor. Based on the commonality of the items, factor 1 is named Talking to One's Partner. Likewise, there are four items that define the second factor—SE1, SE6, SE8, SE10. The common element here seems to be refusal, and the factor is named Refusal. The final factor is defined by items SE2, SE4, SE 9, and SE11 and is named Using a Condom.

To make the factor interpretation easier, it is helpful to use the SPSS Options command to generate a rotated matrix in which the items are ordered by the value of the factor loading (Figure 12.11). In addition, the Suppression command can be used to suppress all values under .10 (default) or a selected value. For the SE scale shown in Table 12.15, we requested that values under .30 be suppressed. Compare the pattern matrix in Table 12.13 to that in Table 12.15 and notice how much easier the pattern matrix in Table 12.15 is to read.

Some authors favor selecting items with factor loadings of .30 (Comrey & Lee, 1992) or .40 or higher (Pett, Lackey, and Sullivan, 2003). In either case, items that have loadings of less than .30 do not share a significant amount of variance with the factor and may be considered for elimination. Other authors (Mulaik, 2004; Preacher & MacCallum, 2003) frown on using an arbitrary cutoff. An item may have a loading of less than .30, but would still be considered important in the interpretation of a factor. They advise the researcher to consider the full range of factor loadings on each factor noting those that have both high and near zero loadings and to report all of the factor loadings in publications for readers to evaluate.

As with the sports activities, we might find that some items that load on a factor are only marginally related to other items on the same factor or might share some similarities with items loading on other factors. For example, water aerobics was included

FIGURE 12.11. SPSS DIALOG BOX FOR THE OPTIONS COMMANDS.

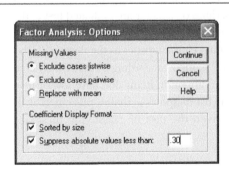

TABLE 12.15. SPSS PRINTOUT OF THE ROTATED PATTERN MATRIX FOR THE 12-ITEM SE SCALE USING THE SORT AND SUPPRESSION COMMANDS UNDER OPTIONS.

Pattern Matrix[a]

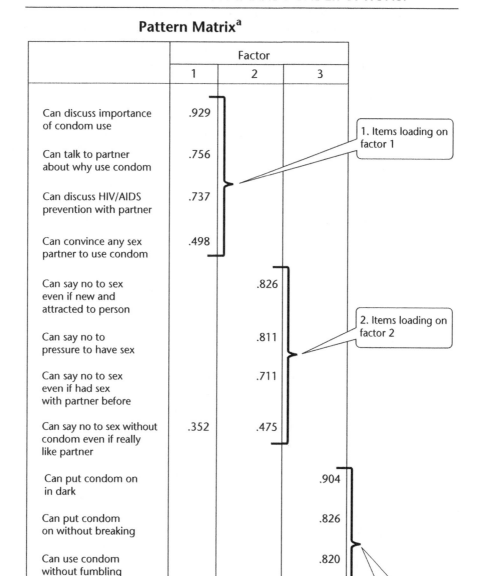

	Factor		
	1	2	3
Can discuss importance of condom use	.929		
Can talk to partner about why use condom	.756		
Can discuss HIV/AIDS prevention with partner	.737		
Can convince any sex partner to use condom	.498		
Can say no to sex even if new and attracted to person		.826	
Can say no to pressure to have sex		.811	
Can say no to sex even if had sex with partner before		.711	
Can say no to sex without condom even if really like partner	.352	.475	
Can put condom on in dark			.904
Can put condom on without breaking			.826
Can use condom without fumbling			.820
Can put condom on even with new partner			.686

1. Items loading on factor 1

2. Items loading on factor 2

3. Items loading on factor 3

Extraction method: maximum likelihood.
Rotation method: Oblimin with Kaiser normalization.
[a]Rotation converged in seven iterations.

under the category of water activities. However, it could also have been placed with aerobics because of the cardiovascular focus of the activity. On the SE scale, the factor loading of SE6 was .352 on factor 1 and .475 on factor 2 suggesting similarities with both factors. Some sets of items express more than one idea, indicating a bimodal, multimodal, or general factor. When this situation occurs, the task of naming factors becomes more difficult. Occasionally, it may not be possible to name a factor. In this situation, Pett, Lackey, and Sullivan (2003) suggest calling it factor 1 (or 2 or 3) until further study helps illuminate its meaning.

If the researcher began with a hypothesis about the number or types of factors, the interpretation process is conducted in light of the theory or hypothesis guiding the analysis. Here, the researcher wants to know whether the factors are consistent with the theory or hypothesis on which the analysis was based. This evaluation has two levels. The researcher evaluates the content of the factors, to determine first whether the constructs underlying the factors are consistent with the theoretical framework, and second, whether the items written to measure each underlying construct actually load on the appropriate factor. With the OE scale for eating a healthy diet, we would expect to extract three factors composed of four items each. One level of evaluation is to determine whether the three factors exist; the other is to determine whether the items written for each dimension actually load on one factor.

If the number or the composition of the factors is not consistent with the hypothesis, the researcher can conduct a second FA and request an analysis that will yield the number of factors originally proposed. The results of this second analysis can be examined to determine whether the structure of the scale is closer to the hypothesized structure. There are no clear or strict guidelines for this evaluation process. Rather, the process is based on clear goals, strong theoretical knowledge, and empirical data derived from the FA. The ideal factor solution is one in which there is correspondence between the predicted and actual numbers of factors composing an instrument and between the predicted and actual placement of items on factors. Unfortunately, this is a rare event even with the most carefully developed instruments. The number of factors may be greater or smaller than the number conceptualized, and items that are thought to measure a factor may load on another factor.

In many factor solutions, there are a few items that have similar loadings on more than one factor. These items are considered cross-loading when the values of the factor loadings differ by less than .20 (or .15) from each other. Cross-loading indicates that the items share characteristics with items on more than one factor, much like water aerobics, which can be placed in the aerobics category or the swimming category. The researcher can do one of several things: (1) place the item on the factor with the highest loading, (2) place the item on the factor with the best conceptual fit, (3) rewrite the item to fit better with items on one factor, or (4) delete the item. Items with loadings of less than .30 (or .40) on all factors are generally deleted. However, Pett, Lackey, and Sullivan (2003) suggest retaining these items if the item is an essential for the scale.

An essential item might function poorly if the item were not relevant for the sample selected for the FA. For example, an item on conflict with spouses might be an important item for an interpersonal-conflict scale. However, if data are collected from mostly single men and women, the item will probably show low factor loading.

Throughout the process, it is important to keep in mind the purpose of the analysis. Conducting the factor analysis to identify the factor structure will lead to one set of decisions, whereas an analysis to identify weak items might lead to another set. Decisions should be consistent with the reason for doing the analysis. A researcher interested in selecting only strong items for each factor might elect to delete cross-loading items, a researcher interested in identifying the factor structure might retain such items, and a researcher interested in shortening a scale might decide to select items from one factor and discard the remaining items.

Confirmatory Factor Analysis

EFA is used to explore the internal structure of the scale. Researchers use EFA to answer questions such as these: How many factors exist in the data? What items are within each factor? Which items are of limited value and can be deleted? Are the number and types of factors consistent with the underlying theoretical framework used in scale development? EFA is often referred to as a form of construct validity and included in the set of tests used to assess the validity of a new scale. EFA is also used to assess the validity of an already developed scale when data are collected from another sample or from another population. In these latter cases, the results of EFA are often compared to the results of the EFA conducted on the original data to evaluate the stability of the factors among different samples or populations.

Confirmatory factor analysis (CFA) is used to validate the relationship among factors and between each item and its factor. CFA is used when the investigator has some prior information about the structure of the scale, usually from a previous EFA. Researchers use CFA to test hypotheses about the relationships among factors and items. CFA can answer questions such as these: Do the proposed number of factors actually exist? Do the items selected for each dimension measure those dimensions? Although it is possible for a researcher to use CFA rather than EFA in the initial validity assessments for a new scale, most researchers first assess the structure of the scale using EFA (Mulaik, 2004). More often than not, EFA suggests items that could be deleted, revised, or added. After revisions, researchers then use CFA to validate the structure using data from another sample. Some researchers use the same techniques described above for EFA as a means of confirming the factor structure. However, structural equation modeling is a more sophisticated, and preferred, technique.

To conduct a CFA, the research begins with a model such as that shown in Figure 12.12, which is the SE scale obtained from EFA. The factors (also called latent

FIGURE 12.12. LATENT VARIABLE MODEL FOR SEM ANALYSIS.

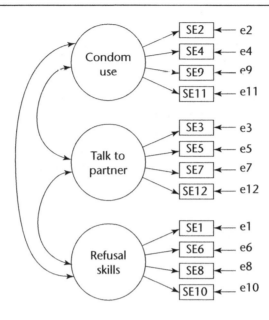

variables) are displayed as circles, and the items (also called indicators or manifest variables) are shown as rectangles. The lines connecting the items to the factors represent correlations between them. Although it is not shown here, owing to the EFA, we know that each line represents different values. Notice also the curved lines connecting the factors. These indicate that there is some correlation among the factors themselves. Also notice the error terms (e_i), one of which is linked to each indicator. There are no lines connecting the error terms to each other, implying that the errors are not correlated.

In CFA, the researcher tests whether the relationships as depicted in the model and the strength of the relationships as determined by previous analysis can be reproduced using the responses of another group of participants. SEM is used to determine whether "the model fits the data." If the correlations and covariances can be reproduced as shown in the model, there is further evidence for the validity of the scale. If the model cannot be reproduced, or only portions of it can be reproduced, the researcher can make modifications in the model and test these modifications using SEM. SEM analyses are complex and require additional study beyond that required to conduct an EFA and interpret the results. Students who are interested in more advanced study in this area should see Bollen (1989), James, Mulaik, and Brett (1982), Mulaik (2003), and Pedhazur and Schmelkin (1991).

Summary

We have devoted this chapter to a fairly detailed discussion of EFA. EFA is used extensively in the health behavior field as a means of assessing the validity of scales. Though the underlying mathematical techniques of factor analysis are complex, statistical software makes it relatively easy for the researcher to conduct a factor analysis. The decisions and the interpretation of the output, however, require an understanding and appreciation of the scale development. EFA analysis can be followed by confirmatory factor analysis, the goal of which is to determine whether the relationships among factors and items arising from EFA can be reproduced using another set of responses to the scale.

CHAPTER THIRTEEN

ITEM RESPONSE THEORY

Frances McCarty

LEARNING OBJECTIVES

At the end of this chapter, the student should be able to

1. Describe some disadvantages related to the use of classical test theory.
2. Describe the basic idea behind item response theory.
3. List and describe the item parameters appearing in common item response theory models.

Classical test theory, or true-score theory, has been and will most likely continue to be used as a framework for the development of tests and instruments. (To simplify the language in this chapter, the term *test* will be used to refer both to traditional knowledge tests and to scales intended to measure other attributes.) Because CTT is based on relatively weak theoretical assumptions, it is applicable in a wide variety of test development situations. Thus, an understanding of the application of CTT to test development will serve the potential test developer well. However, an alternative theory that can be used for test development, item response theory, is increasingly being applied to the development of tests. Whereas CTT focuses primarily on test-level information, IRT, as its name suggests, places more emphasis on item-level information. Although classical test theory does make use of difficulty and discrimination indexes (discussed in Chapter Five) with respect to individual items, the general focus is on the total score (that is, the observed score) and its relationship to the theoretically based true score. Recall that when CTT has been used as the basis for instrument development, one is likely to see a presentation of group-level statistics such as the observed-score mean and standard deviation as well as some measure or measures of reliability (standard error of measurement or an internal consistency, stability, or equivalence coefficient).

Disadvantages of Classical Test Theory

Although CTT has provided a useful theoretical framework for test development, there are several limitations associated with its use. One frequently cited limitation of CTT, and very likely the most important one, is the dependent relationship found between the person and item statistics. One translation of this is that the item statistics (that is, difficulty and discrimination) are sample dependent (dependent on the group that has taken the test) and the person statistic (observed score for a person) is item sample dependent. A second translation is that the item difficulty and discrimination values obtained are dependent on the ability level of the group taking the test and the observed score for a person is dependent on the particular set of items presented to that person. For example, the difficulty values obtained for the items on a math test may indicate that the items are all relatively easy if most of the students taking the test have *high* math ability. However, if we give the same set of test items to a group of students identified as having *low* math ability, we may find that the difficulty values obtained are indicative of items that are relatively difficult. In terms of the person statistic, suppose we are interested in measuring a person's math ability and we develop two tests, one with 75 percent of the items considered *easy* (test A) and one with 75 percent of the items considered *difficult* (test B). Further, let us suppose that a person of *average* math ability takes both test A and test B, scoring 95 and 65, respectively. If we look at the person's observed score on test A (the easy test), we may conclude that this person, known to have *average* math ability, has *high* math ability. However, if we look at the person's observed score on test B (the difficult test), we may come to the conclusion that the person actually has *low* math ability. In this case, the person's observed score depends on the sample of items presented.

Along with the problem of dependent person and item statistics, CTT has some other limiting aspects. Recall that the standard error of measurement can be used as one way of quantifying the reliability of a test. From a practical standpoint, a single standard error of measurement is obtained and used to create a confidence interval around individual predicted true scores, giving an indication of precision at the level of the individual test taker. The problem with this approach is that one standard error of measurement is applied to all observed objects of measurement (persons) despite the fact that it may not be reasonable to assume that the amount of error is constant across the continuum of the characteristic being measured. Generally, the level of precision is less for more extreme observations (that is, individuals with very low or very high levels of a characteristic).

Because CTT is really a *test-based* theory as opposed to an *item-based* theory, there are also some more practical limitations associated with its use. The true-score model that serves as the basis for much of CTT does not provide a way of determining how a person or group may perform on any one particular item. This limitation has important implications for the interpretation of test scores and the development of tests that meet specific design criteria.

As one might imagine, we have presented a discussion of the disadvantages of CTT as the framework for test development as a way of introducing the idea that item response theory, when appropriately applied, can overcome some of these disadvantages. From a theoretical standpoint, IRT overcomes the major limitation of CTT by producing person and item statistics that are not dependent on the set of items administered or the group that has taken the test. This property is referred to as the invariance property; it is the property that allows IRT to overcome many of the limitations associated with CTT. The invariance property has important implications for the comparison of scores on the same test across different test-taking groups as well as comparison of scores on different forms of a test. Unlike scores obtained from a classical theory framework, which would make these types of comparisons impossible, scores obtained using IRT methods do allow such comparisons, facilitating applications such as test equating and computer-adapted testing.

In addition to the advantages provided by the invariance property inherent in IRT models, these models also provide a means for estimating separate standard errors across the continuum of ability. In other words, we are not constrained by a single standard error of measurement that must be applied to all objects of measurement (persons). This is an important advantage, given that precision is not considered to be constant across the range of ability.

A number of authors (see Hambleton, Swaminathan, & Rogers, 1991; Hambleton & Jones, 1993; or Fan, 1998) provide a good introduction to the advantages of using IRT and provide a more thorough comparison of IRT and classical test theory.

Item Response Theory Basics

Before we move on to the basics of IRT, a brief discussion of terminology may alleviate some of the confusion that is often encountered when IRT concepts are presented. In fact, you may have already experienced this confusion in the preceding discussion. First, an item may be defined as a single, individual indicator, or measure, of a particular characteristic. Moving up the hierarchy, there are three terms that are often used interchangeably to describe a collection of items intended to measure a particular characteristic: *test, scale,* and *instrument.* Whereas the term *test* is most often used in the context of educational measurement, the terms *scale* and *instrument* are more likely to appear in the context of psychosocial measurement. As we mentioned earlier, the term *test* will be used throughout the following discussion to introduce a degree of consistency.

Up to this point, we have consistently made references to some *characteristic* that is being measured. In fact, several terms are often used interchangeably to refer to the characteristic that is being measured by a collection of items. The following terms are all used to refer to this latent characteristic of interest: *trait, ability,* and *theta.* The implication of the latent component of that definition is directly related to the idea that some underlying, unobservable characteristic influences an individual's response to any one item. Consider math ability. Though we cannot directly observe an individual's underlying math ability, we would expect that individual's math ability to influence his or her responses to a collection of items intended to measure math ability. Thus, someone whose latent math ability is high would be expected to respond one way (answer correctly), whereas someone whose latent math ability is low would be expected to respond another way (answer incorrectly). Depending on the characteristic being measured, one of the three terms may make the most conceptual sense. For example, the term *ability* fits well in the context of educational measurement, whereas *trait* may fit better in the context of psychosocial measurement. The term *theta*, often indicated by a lowercase Greek letter (θ), could be considered a more generic term and tends to be used in theoretical or mathematical presentations of IRT.

The IRT framework for test development encompasses a group, or family, of models that can be applied to a variety of testing situations. The particular model employed depends on the nature of the test items and on whether certain theoretical assumptions can be made about the test. In terms of the nature of the test items, a number of models have been developed that are applicable to dichotomously scored items—for example, *correct/incorrect.* As one might guess, these particular models have been applied and studied extensively in the context of educational testing situations, where correct/incorrect scoring is prevalent. However, one should note that these models may be equally valid for other dichotomous scoring schemes—for example, *presence/absence.* In addition to the more widely applied dichotomous models, a variety of polytomous item response models have been developed to capture the information obtained when more than two categories are available to score a given item. Specifically, polytomous IRT models are useful when responses are collected using a Likert-type format. These models are especially applicable to the development of tests created to measure psychosocial traits, because many of these measures use scoring schemes that include more than two options.

In terms of the theoretical assumptions that go along with the application of item response models, the most important is related to the dimensionality of the test. Many of the widely applied IRT models make the assumption that the test is unidimensional. In other words, they assume that the set of items measures one and only one ability or trait and that an individual's response to any one item is a function of that one ability or trait. Strictly speaking, this assumption is rarely met, because a number of factors other than the trait under consideration are likely to have some influence on an individual's performance on a test. This being the case, in practice, the unidimensionality assumption is considered a viable assumption when a single and dominant component or factor is deemed sufficient to account for performance on the set of items. Multidimensional models have been developed for situations in which the unidimensionality assumption is clearly not reasonable. These models are fairly complicated and have not been widely applied in practice. Because this is the case, the following discussion of IRT will focus on the more widely applied unidimensional models.

To fully understand the more technical aspects of IRT, it is important to keep in mind that IRT models are intended to provide a link between responses to a set of items and a latent characteristic that is not directly observable. The main focus of IRT is to use observed behavior (responses to a set of items) to estimate an individual's standing on some latent characteristic. When we apply IRT models in practical situations, we are making the assumption that the probability of seeing a particular type of response or behavior is related to the person's standing on the underlying trait of interest.

At this point, it may be helpful to think about two different testing situations, one focusing on a test of general nutrition knowledge and the other focusing on a scale intended to measure test anxiety. The items and response options for the two hypothetical tests are presented in Table 13.1. In the case of the general nutrition test, whose items are scored correct/incorrect, the probability of a correct response to any one item is stated as a function of the hypothesized latent characteristic, general nutrition knowledge. An individual with a high level of nutrition knowledge would correspondingly have a higher probability of answering correctly. In the case of the test anxiety scale, which has four response options, the probability of responding in a higher category (for example, the *agree* category) is expressed as a function of the latent characteristic, test anxiety. An individual with a high level of test anxiety would have a higher probability of responding in the upper categories (strongly agree, agree) than would an individual with a low level of test anxiety.

Although it might be agreeable to continue the discussion of IRT without moving into the world of mathematical formulas, this may be a good point to begin a brief discussion of the more technical aspects of IRT models. The foundation of IRT models is the item characteristic curve, also referred to as an item characteristic function or an item response function. An ICC is a monotonically increasing function that describes the relationship between the level of an underlying trait and performance on an item. In the case of dichotomously scored items, the function specifies that as the underlying-trait level increases, the probability of a correct response to an item increases. The *S*-shaped curve shown in Figure 13.1 is an example of an item characteristic curve.

TABLE 13.1. ITEMS FOR TWO HYPOTHETICAL TESTS.

General Nutrition Knowledge	Response Options
1. Carbohydrates, proteins, and fats all provide four calories per gram. (False)	True or False, scored as Correct (0) or Incorrect (1) using the provided key.
2. The current food pyramid consists of five food groups. (True)	
3. Vegetarian diets are never consistent with recommended dietary guidelines. (False).	
4. Fiber is found only in plant foods. (True.)	
5. A certain amount of dietary fat is needed for good health. (True.)	

Test Anxiety	
1. I become physically ill when I have to take a test.	Strongly agree, Agree, Disagree, or Strongly disagree, scored as 4, 3, 2, 1, respectively.
2. I experience a great deal of apprehension when I have to take a test.	
3. I become anxious in the minutes before a test is scheduled to begin.	
4. I experience increasing amounts of anxiety as I progress through the test period.	
5. I get nervous when I think about taking a test	

FIGURE 13.1. EXAMPLE OF AN ITEM CHARACTERISTIC CURVE.

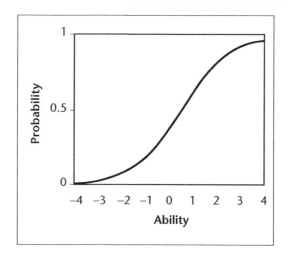

As we have stated, a number of item response models can be used with unidimensional tests. The different models are characterized by the mathematical form of the ICC or the number of item parameters included in the model, or both. Item parameters are simply values used to specify the actual characteristics of an item. These specific values will determine the actual appearance of the ICC. As we will discuss below, difficulty, discrimination, and pseudo-chance parameters are the item characteristics used in common IRT models.

Three common models are used when a test is unidimensional and scored in a dichotomous fashion. These models are relatively easy to remember because they are referred to in terms of the number of parameters used to describe the item characteristic curve. As we have mentioned, there are three item parameters that can appear in the most common models: (1) an item discrimination, or a, parameter, (2) an item difficulty, or b, parameter, and (3) a pseudo-chance, or c, parameter. The simplest and most widely used model is the one-parameter logistic model, which includes only a difficulty (or b) parameter; the discrimination (or a) parameter is considered to be the same across all items on the test; and the c parameter is set to 0, suggesting that those with the lowest ability levels will have a zero probability of responding correctly. The two-parameter logistic model includes the a and b parameters. Finally, as you might expect, the three-parameter logistic model includes all three item parameters, a, b, and c. In the three-parameter model, the c parameter allows the lower asymptote of the ICC to take on a value greater than 0, suggesting that even those at the lowest ability levels have a probability greater than 0 of responding correctly to a given item. The equations for the ICCs for the one-, two-, and three-parameter logistic models are given in Exhibit 13.1. When models are applied in practice, the simplest model that fits the data is usually chosen. In other words, the addition of either the a or the c parameter would occur only if it produced an improvement in the model-data fit.

The interpretation of the item parameters is fairly straightforward. The value of the b, or item difficulty, parameter can be found at the point of inflection on the item characteristic curve, and for the one- and two- parameter models is the place on the ability scale at which a test taker has a .50 probability of responding correctly. For the three-parameter model, it is the point at which the probability of responding correctly is $(1 + c)/2$. Higher values of b are indicative of greater item difficulty, with values generally ranging from -2 to $+2$. Conveniently, the difficulty and ability (theta) values are normally expressed on the same scale. Therefore, for the one- and two-parameter models, if the value of b_i is .5, the following interpretation can be made: a randomly chosen test taker whose ability level (theta) is equal to .5 will have a .5 probability of responding correctly to the given item.

The a parameter—included in the two- and three-parameter models—adds an additional piece of information about the item. The value of a can range from $-\infty$ to $+\infty$ and is proportional to the slope of the ICC at the point of inflection on the

EXHIBIT 13.1. EQUATIONS FOR THE ONE-, TWO-, AND THREE-PARAMETER LOGISTIC IRT MODELS.

One-Parameter Model	Two-Parameter Model	Three-Parameter Model
$i = 1, 2, \ldots n$	$i = 1, 2, \ldots n$	$i = 1, 2, \ldots n$

where

$P_i(\theta)$ = probability that a randomly chosen object of measurement (person) with ability theta (θ) answers item i correctly; when taken over the range of the ability scale, will result in an S-shaped curve with values between 0 and 1.

b_i = difficulty parameter for item i.

a_i = discrimination parameter for item i.

c_i = lower asymptote (pseudo-chance) parameter for item i.

n = number of items in the test, and

D = scaling factor equal to 1.7.

ability scale. Items with steeper slopes do a better job of discriminating among test takers of high and low ability. Very low values of a indicate that an item discriminates poorly, and negative values would be indicative of a very problematic item.

Finally, the c parameter—included in the three-parameter model—allows the lower asymptote of the ICC to take on a value greater than 0. In the one- and two-parameter models, the lower asymptote of the ICC will reflect the fact that those at the lowest level of the ability continuum will have a zero probability of responding correctly to a given item. The addition of the c parameter essentially lifts this probability so that even those at the lowest level will have a greater-than-zero probability of responding correctly to the given item. The inclusion of a c parameter is often applied to tests with multiple-choice items, tests in which even those at the low end of the ability range may be able to employ guessing methods that lead to correct response choices.

To better understand how the item parameters function, it is helpful to look at some theoretical ICCs based on the three different models. Figure 13.2 depicts ICCs for the one-, two-, and three-parameter models for four different items. For the one-parameter model, note that the curves all look very similar except for the left-to-right shifting, which indicates differing levels of difficulty for the four items. Item 1 is the least difficult; the value of the b parameter is equal to −.5, which indicates that test takers at −.5 on the ability scale have about a 50 percent chance of responding correctly. If you look at item 4, which is the most difficult, you can see that those same test takers, those at −.5 on the ability scale, have a relatively small chance (about 10 percent) of responding correctly to item 4. According to this model, only test takers whose ability level is greater than or equal to 1.5 will have a 50 percent or better chance of responding correctly. If you look at the graph for the two-parameter model, you can see that items 1 and 2 have the same discrimination parameter but different difficulty parameters. However, if you look at items 3 and 4, you will note that the difficulty values are the same but the discrimination values are different. In this case, item 4 does a better job than item 3 of discriminating between those at the upper and lower ends of the ability range. In the final graph, depicting items using a three-parameter model, you can see that the lower ends (asymptotes) of three of the four curves rise above the value of 0, indicating that even those with very low ability have a greater-than-zero chance of responding correctly. Interpretation of the *a* and *b* parameters is similar to that previously described for the two-parameter model. Remember, however, that the interpretation of *b* is slightly different. For the three-parameter model, *b* is interpreted as the location on the ability continuum at which the probability of responding correctly is equal to $(1 + c)/2$. For item 1, a test taker with an ability of −1 would have about a 60 percent chance of responding correctly to item 1.

FIGURE 13.2. THEORETICAL ICCS FOR ONE-, TWO-, AND THREE-PARAMETER LOGISTIC IRT MODELS FOR FOUR ITEMS WITH GIVEN PARAMETER VALUES.

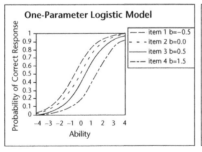

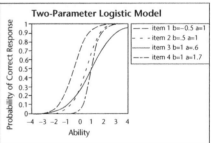

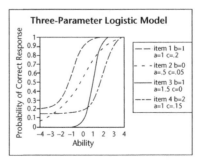

Polytomous Models

As mentioned earlier, polytomous item response models are available for use when more than two response categories are used to score an item. Because many instruments developed to measure health behaviors use a Likert-type response format, a brief introduction to polytomous IRT models is presented.

A number of models have been developed to handle polytomous response formats. One of these models is Samejima's graded response (GR) model. This particular model is appropriate when the items under consideration have response options that are successively ordered. For example, an instrument designed to measure the frequency of a certain type of behavior may offer never, sometimes, or always as the response options. In the GR model, the graded scoring of an item is approached from a boundary or threshold perspective. In other words, there is a boundary above which a person is expected to obtain certain category scores as opposed to lower category scores. For example, if there are three categories denoted as 0 (never), 1 (sometimes), and 2 (always), the focus is on the probability of obtaining scores of 1 or 2 versus 0, or the probability of obtaining a score of 2 versus scores of 0 or 1. With the GR model the more steps that are successfully completed, in this example 0, 1, or 2, the larger the category score, which is indicative of a higher level of the trait (De Ayala, 1993).

The GR model specifies the probability of a person responding in category k or higher as opposed to responding in categories lower than k. Responses to item i are categorized into $m_i + 1$ categories, where m_i is the number of category boundaries for item i and higher categories indicate greater ability or a higher level of a particular trait. Each category of item i has a category score, x_i, with integer values 0, 1 . . . m_i. Similar to the equations presented in Exhibit 13.1, the respondent-item interaction is modeled as

$$P_{ik}^+(\theta) = \frac{\exp\left[Da_i(\theta_s - b_{ik})\right]}{1 + \exp\left[Da_i(\theta_s - b_{ik})\right]}$$

where θ is the latent trait, D is a scaling constant equal to 1.702, b_{ik} is the difficulty parameter for category k for item I, and a_i is the discrimination parameter for item i. In the most common case of the graded response model it is assumed that a_i is constant within an item across thresholds, but not necessarily across items. That is, the category characteristic curves (CCC) have equal slopes for each category in an item, which means that the curves within an item will not cross. In terms of the difficulty parameter, multiple b-parameters are required such that the number of b-parameters is equal to the number of categories in an item minus one. For our *never, sometimes, and always* response category example, there would be two b-parameters (3 response categories-1) per item.

Similar to the item characteristic curve presented in Figure 13.1, Figure 13.3 shows a category characteristic curve (CCC) or boundary response function (BRF) for a three-category item. In this case, the respondent could receive a score of 0, 1, or 2. The CCCs depicted here are for an item with $a = 1.5$, $b_1 = -1.0$, and $b_2 = 1.0$. The first curve (labeled 1) represents the probability of scoring at or above 1. The second curve represents the probability of scoring at or above 2.

In order to obtain the probability of responding in a particular category, the difference between the cumulative probabilities for adjacent categories is calculated. Mathematically, this is represented by

$$P_{ik}(\theta) = P_{ik}^{+}(\theta) - P_{i,k+1}^{+}(\theta)$$

This function is referred to as the item category response function (ICRF). The number of response functions per item corresponds to the number of response categories. In order to calculate the first and last categories, a modification must be made to

FIGURE 13.3. CCC FOR A THREE-CATEGORY GRADED RESPONSE MODEL WHERE $A = 1.5$, $B_1 = -1.0$, AND $B_2 = 1.0$.

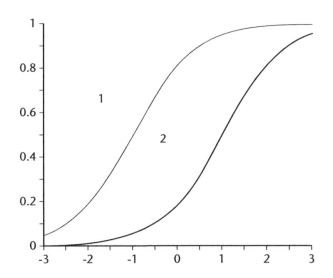

account for the lack of an adjacent category. In the case of responding in the first category on item i, the probability is expressed as

$$P_{i1}(\theta) = 1 - P_{ik}^{+}(\theta)$$

The probability of responding in the last category for item i is

$$P_{ik}(\theta) = P_{i,k-1}^{+}(\theta) - 0$$

Figure 13.4 shows the item category response functions (ICRFs) for a three-category item. The ICRFs are interpreted from left to right and represent the probability of scoring 0 (never), 1 (sometimes), or 2 (always), respectively. Specifically, the fine dotted line represents the probability of obtaining a category score of 0, the solid line represents the probability of obtaining a category score of 1, and the heavy dotted

FIGURE13.4. ICRFS FOR A THREE-CATEGORY ITEM
WHERE $A = 1.5$, $B_1 = -1$, AND $B_2 = 1$.

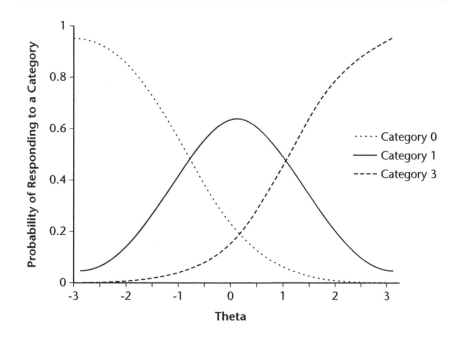

line presents the probability of obtaining a category score of 2, all given theta. From a practical standpoint, the ICRFs enable one to readily see the probability that a particular category will be chosen or endorsed given the trait level of the respondent. For example, in Figure 13.4, a randomly selected respondent who has a theta value (trait level) of 2 has an extremely low probability of choosing category 0, a small probability of choosing category 1, and a relatively high probability of choosing category 3.

Technical Issues

At this point, you may be wondering how item parameter and ability values are obtained. Similar to the way tests are developed using the CTT framework, a test is administered to a group of test takers (*examinees* in the jargon of educational measurement), and their item responses on the test are subjected to analysis, using specialized software. In actual applications, both the item parameters and the ability parameters are estimated, using the examinees' responses to the items on the test of interest. Without going into technical details, these estimations involve an iterative process in which information from one is incorporated into the estimation of the other. This process is what leads to the invariance property discussed earlier in this chapter. On a technical note, most IRT software packages employ maximum likelihood–based procedures to estimate item and examinee parameters. Several factors contribute to the accuracy of estimates obtained. As with other procedures that invoke some type of mathematical modeling, the appropriateness of the model chosen to model the data can have an important impact on the accuracy of the estimates. Obviously, if the chosen model fits the data well, the obtained estimates are likely to be more accurate. Other factors contributing to the accuracy of the estimates include the number of parameters that must be estimated (fewer is usually better), the number of items on the test and the number of examinees included (more is usually better), and finally, the dimensionality of the data. As we have discussed, the more readily applied models (including the ones presented in this chapter) tend to make the assumption that the test items are measuring a single latent characteristic (unidimensionality). If a unidimensional model is applied to a multidimensional test, the estimates will to some extent be adversely affected.

As we noted at the beginning of this chapter, IRT methods have the potential to overcome the major limitation associated with CTT (dependency that is present in person and item statistics). Although this is seen as the major advantage of IRT, the additional item information obtained from IRT analyses may be a more important advantage, because this information can be used to construct tests that include the best items for a given testing purpose.

Like all methods that seem to provide a "quick fix," IRT methods should be used cautiously, giving due consideration to the appropriateness of the model, the number of items on the test, the number of examinees in the sample, and the ultimate purpose of the test. Traditionally, sample size (that is, the number of examinees) has been a serious limiting factor in terms of the actual application of IRT models to real data. As noted in our brief discussion of parameter estimation, larger sample sizes are desirable; the traditional minimum recommendation is 500 examinees. Although the methods can be applied to relatively small samples (say, 100 in the case of a one-parameter model), item-parameter and ability estimates may be less accurate and will need to be interpreted with caution. When IRT methods are being used in the initial test development phase to identify potential test items from a pool, smaller sample sizes may be less of a concern. However, if the desire is to obtain final item parameters that will be used in the scoring and reporting of an IRT-based standardized test, the importance of an adequate sample (in terms of size and examinee characteristics) cannot be overemphasized.

Summary

The information included in this chapter is intended to give the reader a basic introduction to IRT. Although IRT models have traditionally been used to develop large-scale standardized achievement and aptitude tests, IRT models are increasingly being used to develop tests intended to measure psychosocial constructs. This being the case, it has become more important that those involved in measurement-related activities have at least some basic knowledge of IRT.

For those who would like to fill in the many gaps left by this chapter, one of the following references would be appropriate: Hambleton, Swaminathan, and Rogers (1991), Hulin, Drasgow, and Parsons (1983), and Embretson and Reise (2000). In addition, the following articles provide more thorough introductions to some of the topics presented in this chapter: Harris (1989), Hambleton and Jones (1993), Fan (1998), and De Ayala (1993).

REFERENCES

AARDEX, Ltd. (2005). Retrieved from http://www.aardex.ch

Ajzen, I. (1991). The theory of planned behavior. *Organizational Behavior and Human Decision Processes, 50,* 179–211.

American Educational Research Association, American Psychological Association, and National Council on Measurement in Education. (1999). *Standards for educational and psychological testing.* Washington, DC: American Educational Research Association.

Bandura, A. (1997). *Self-efficacy: The exercise of control.* New York: Freeman.

Bassey, E. J., Dallosso, H. M., et al. (1987). Validation of a simple mechanical accelerometer (pedometer) for the estimation of walking activity. *European Journal of Applied Physiology and Occupational Physiology, 56,* 323–330.

Binet, A., & Simon, T. (1973). *The development of intelligence in children: The Binet-Simon scale.* New York: Arno.

Bloom, B. S. (Ed.). (1956). *Taxonomy of educational objectives: The classification of educational goals. Handbook I: Cognitive domain.* New York: Longmans, Green.

Bollen, K. (1989). *Structural equations modeling with latent variables.* New York: Wiley.

Bollen, K., & Lennox, R. (1991). Conventional wisdom on measurement: A structural equation perspective. *Psychological Bulletin, 110*(2), 305–314.

Brennan, R. L. (2001). *Generalizability theory.* New York: Springer.

Brown, W. (1910). Some experimental results in the correlation of mental abilities. *British Journal of Psychology, 3*(3), 296–322.

Bullen, P., & Onyx, J. (2005). Measuring social capital in five communities in NSW. Retrieved from http://www.mapl.com.au/A2htm

Camilli, G., & Shepard, L. A. (1994). *Methods for identifying biased test items.* Thousand Oaks, CA: Sage.

Campbell, D. T., & Fiske, D. W. (1959). Convergent and discriminant validation by the multitrait-multimethod matrix. *Psychological Bulletin, 56*(2), 81–105.

Campbell, D. T., & Russo, M. J. (2001). *Social measurement.* Thousand Oaks, CA: Sage.

Carmines, E. G., & Zeller, R. A. (1979). *Reliability and validity assessment.* Thousand Oaks, CA: Sage.

Cattell, R. B. (1966). The scree test for the number of factors. *Multivariate Behavioral Research, 1*, 245–276.

Chesney, M. A., Ickovics, J. R., et al. (2000). Self-reported adherence to antiretroviral medications among participants in HIV clinical trials: The AACTG adherence instruments (Patient Care Committee and Adherence Working Group of the Outcomes Committee of the Adult AIDS Clinical Trials Group [AACTG]). *AIDS Care, 12*(3), 255–266.

Chinn, P. L., & Kramer, M. K. (1995). *Theory and nursing: A systematic approach.* St. Louis: Mosby.

Clark, H. H., & Schober, M. F. (1994). Asking questions and influencing answers. In J. M. Tanur (Ed.), *Questions about questions: Inquiries into the cognitive bases of surveys* (pp. 15–48). New York, Russell Sage Foundation.

Cline, M. E., Herman, J., et al. (1992). Standardization of the visual analogue scale. *Nursing Research, 41*(6), 378–380.

Cohen, J. (1960). A coefficient of agreement for nominal scales. *Educational and Psychological Measurement, 20*(1), 37–46.

Comrey, A. L., & Lee, H. B. (1992). *A first course in factor analysis.* Mahwah, NJ: Erlbaum.

Cooper, W. H. (1981). Ubiquitous halo. *Psychological Bulletin, 90*(2), 218–244.

Couch, A., & Keniston, K. (1960). Yeasayers and naysayers: Agreeing response set as a personality variable. *Journal of Abnormal and Social Psychology, 60*(2), 151–174.

Cramer, J. A., Mattson, R. H., et al. (1989). How often is medication taken as prescribed? A novel assessment technique. *JAMA, 261*, 3273–3277.

Crane, G. R. (Ed.). (2004). Perseus Digital Library Project. Tufts University. Retrieved from http://www.perseus.tufts.edu

Crick, J. E., & Brennan, R. L. (1983). *Manual for GENOVA: A generalized analysis of variance systems.* Iowa City, IA: American College Testing Program.

Crocker, L., & Algina, J. (1986). *Introduction to classical and modern test theory.* Orlando: Harcourt Brace.

Cronbach, L. J. (1946). Response sets and test validity. *Educational and Psychological Measurement, 6*, 475–494.

Cronbach, L. J. (1951). Coefficient alpha and the internal structure of tests. *Psychometrika, 16*(3), 297–334.

Cronbach, L. J., & Meehl, P. E. (1955). Construct validity in psychological tests. *Psychological Bulletin, 52*(4), 281–302.

Cronbach, L. J., Rajaratnam, N., & Gleser, G. C. (1963). Theory of generalizability: A liberalization of reliability theory. *British Journal of Statistical Psychology, 16* (pt. 2), 137–163.

Cronk, B. C. (1999). *How to use SPSS: A step-by-step guide to analysis and interpretation.* Los Angeles: Pyrczak.

Crowne, D. P., & Marlowe, D. (1960). A new scale of social desirability independent of psychopathology. *Journal of Consulting Psychology, 24*(4), 349–354.

Decker, M. D., Booth, A. L., et al. (1986). Validity of food consumption histories in a foodborne outbreak investigation. *American Journal of Epidemiology, 124*(5), 859–863.

De Ayala, R. J. (1993). An introduction to polytomous item response theory models. *Measurement & Evaluation in Counseling & Development, 25*(4), 172–189.

DeVellis, R. F. (2003). *Scale Development: Theory and applications* (2nd ed.). Thousand Oaks, CA: Sage.

Di Iorio, C., et al. (2003). The association of stigma with self-management and perceptions of health care among adults with epilepsy. *Epilepsy and Behavior, 4*(3), 259-267.

Dillman, D. A. (2000). *Mail and Internet surveys: The tailored design method.* New York: Wiley.

DuBois, P. H. (1970). *A history of psychological testing.* Boston: Allyn & Bacon.

Dulock, H. L., & Holzemer, W. L. (1991). Substruction: Improving the linkage from theory to method. *Nursing Science Quarterly, 4*(2), 83–87.

Ebel, R. L. (1965). *Measuring educational achievement.* Upper Saddle River, NJ: Prentice-Hall.

Edwards, A. L. (1957). *The social desirability variable in personality assessment research.* Orlando: Dryden Press.

Embretson, S., & Reise, S. (2000). *Item response theory for psychologists.* Mahway, NJ: Erlbaum.

Emerson, R. M. (1976). Social exchange theory. *Annual Review of Sociology, 2,* 335–362.

Erdos, P. L. (1970). *Professional mail surveys.* New York: McGraw-Hill.

Fan, X. (1998). Item response theory and classical test theory: An empirical comparison of their item/person statistics. *Educational & Psychological Measurement, 58*(3), 357-381.

Favre, O., Delacretaz, E., et al. (1997). Relationship between the prescriber's instructions and compliance with antibiotherapy in outpatients treated for acute infectious disease. *Journal of Clinical Pharmacology, 37,* 175–178.

Fishbein, M., & Ajzen, I. (1975). *Belief, attitude, attention, and behavior: An introduction to theory and research.* Reading, MA: Addison-Wesley.

Fisher, R., & Quigley, K. (1992). Applying cognitive theory in public health investigations: Enhancing food recall with the cognitive interview. In J. M. Tanur (Ed.), *Questions about questions: Inquiries into the cognition bases of surveys* (pp. 154–169). New York: Russell Sage Foundation.

Fiske, D. W., & Campbell, D. T. (1992). Citations do not solve problems. *Psychological Bulletin, 112,* 393–395.

Fitts, W. H. (1991). *Tennessee self-concept scale, manual.* Los Angeles: Western Psychological Services.

Freyd, M. (1922). The measurement of interests in vocational selection. *Journal of Personnel Research, 1,* 319–328.

Freyd, M. (1923). The graphic rating scale. *Journal of Educational Psychology, 14,* 83–102.

Gaston-Johansson, F., Fridh, G., & Turner-Norvell, K. (1988). Progression of labor pain in primiparas and multiparas. *Nursing Research, 37*(2), 86–90.

Gibbs, J. P. (1972). *Sociological theory construction.* Orlando: Dryden Press.

Green, S. B., Lissitz, R. W., & Mulaik, S. A. (1977). Limitations of coefficient alpha as an index of test unidimensionality. *Educational and Psychological Measurement, 37,* 827–838.

Gronlund, N. E. (1977). *Constructing achievement tests.* Upper Saddle River, NJ: Prentice-Hall.

Gronlund, N. E. (1978). *Stating objectives for classroom instruction.* New York: Macmillan.

Guttman, L. (1944). A basis for scaling qualitative data. *American Sociological Review, 9*(2), 139–150.

Guttman, L. (1954). Some necessary conditions for common-factor analysis. *Psychometrika, 19*(2), 149–161.

Hambleton, R .K. (1989). Principles and selected applications of item response theory. In R. L. Linn (Ed.), *Educational measurement* (3rd ed.) (pp.147-200). New York: Macmillan.

Hambleton, R. K., & Jones, R. W. (1993). Comparison of classical test theory and item response theory and their applications to test development. *Educational Measurement: Issues & Practice, 12*(3), 38-47.

Hambleton, R. K., Swaminathan, H., & Rogers, H. J. (1991). *Fundamentals of item response theory.* Newbury Park, CA: Sage.

Hambleton, R. K., Swaminathan, H., Algina, J., & Coulson, D. B. (1978). Criterion-referenced testing and measurement: A review of technical issues and developments. *Review of Educational Research, 48*(1), 1–47.

Harris, D. (1989). Comparison of 1-, 2-, and 3- parameter IRT models. *Educational Measurement: Issues & Practice*, Spring, 35-41.

Hulin, C. L., Drasgow, F., & Parsons, C. K. (1983*). Item response theory: Application to psychological measurement.* Homewood, IL: Dow Jones-Irwin.

James, L. R., Mulaik, S. A., & Brett, J. M. (1982). *Causal analysis: Assumptions, models, and data.* Thousand Oaks, CA: Sage.

Jones, R. (2003). Survey data collection using audio computer assisted self-interview. *Western Journal of Nursing Research, 25*(3), 349–358.

Jöreskog, K. G. (1969). A general approach to confirmatory maximum likelihood factor analysis. *Psychometrika, 34*(2), 183–202.

Kaiser, H. F. (1960). The application of electronic computers to factor analysis. *Educational Psychological Measurement, 20*, 141–151.

Kashiwazaki, H., Inaoka, T., et al. (1986). Correlations of pedometer readings with energy expenditure in workers during free-living daily activities. *European Journal of Applied Physiology and Occupational Physiology, 54*, 585–590.

Kerlinger, F. N., & Lee, H. B. (2000). *Foundations of behavioral research* (4th ed.). Northridge, CA: Wadsworth Thomson Learning.

Kleinbaum, D. G., Kupper, L. L., Muller, K. E., & Nizam, A. (1997). *Applied regression analysis and other multivariable methods.* Pacific Grove, CA: Duxbury Press.

Kline, P. (1994). *An easy guide to factor analysis.* New York: Routledge.

Krosnick, J. A. (1991). Response strategies for coping with the cognitive demands of attitude measures in surveys. *Applied Cognitive Psychology, 5*, 213–236.

Kuder, G. F., & Richardson, M. W. (1937). The theory of the estimation of test reliability. *Psychometrika, 2*(3), 151–160.

Landis, J. R., & Koch, G. G. (1977). The measurement of observer agreement for categorical data. *Biometrics, 33*, 159–174.

Lazarus, R. S., & Folkman, S. (1984). *Stress, appraisal, and coping.* New York: Springer.

Likert, R. (1932). A technique for the measurement of attitudes. *Archives of Psychology, 22*(140), 5–55.

Linden, W. J., van der, & Hambleton, R. K. (Eds.). (1997). *Handbook of modern item response theory.* New York: Springer.

Lodge, M. (1981). *Magnitude scaling: Quantitative measurement of opinions.* Thousand Oaks, CA: Sage.

Lord, F. M. (1953). The relation of test score to the trait underlying the test. *Educational and Psychological Measurement, 13*, 517–549.

Lord, F. M., & Novick, M. R. (1968). *Statistical theories of mental test scores.* Reading, MA: Addison-Wesley.

Lowe, T. R. (1986). Eight ways to ruin a performance review. *Personnel Journal, 65*(1), 60–62.

Lynn, M. R. (1986). Determination and quantification of content validity. *Nursing Research, 35*(6), 382–385.

Mangione, T. W. (1995). *Mail surveys: Improving the quality.* Thousand Oaks, CA: Sage.

Mann, J. M. (1981). A prospective study of response error in food history questionnaires: Implications for foodborne outbreak investigation. *American Journal of Public Health 71*, 1362–1366.

Messick, S. (1989). Validity. In R. Linn (Ed.), *Educational measurement* (3rd ed.) (pp. 13–103). New York: Macmillan.

Metzger, D. (2000). Randomized controlled trial of audio computer-assisted self-interviewing: Utility and acceptability in longitudinal studies. *American Journal of Epidemiology, 152*(2), 99–106.

Michell, J. (1990). *An introduction to the logic of psychological measurement.* Mahwah, NJ: Erlbaum.

Mulaik, S. A. (1972). *The foundations of factor analysis.* New York: McGraw-Hill.

Mulaik, S. A. (1987). A brief history of the philosophical foundations of exploratory factor analysis. *Multivariate Behavioral Research, 22*, 267-305.

Mulaik, S. A. (1990). Blurring the distinctions between component analysis and common factor analysis. *Multivariate Behavioral Research, 25*(1), 53-59.

Mulaik, S. A. (2003). Factor analysis. In M. Lewis-Beck, A. E. Bryman, & T. F. Liao (Eds.), *The Sage encyclopedia of social science research methods.* Thousand Oaks, CA: Sage.

Mulaik, S. A. (2004). Objectivity in science and structural equation modeling. In D. Kaplan (Ed.), *The Sage handbook of quantitative methodology for the social sciences* (pp. 423-444). Thousand Oaks, CA: Sage.

Norman, G. R., & Streiner, D. L. (2000). *Biostatistics: The bare essentials.* London: B.C. Decker.

Nunnally, J. C., & Bernstein, I. H. (1994). *Psychometric theory.* New York: McGraw-Hill.

Osgood, C. E. (1952). The nature and measurement of meaning. *Psychological Bulletin, 49*(3), 197–237.

Osterlind, S. J. (1998). *Constructing test items: Multiple-choice, constructed-response, performance, and other formats.* Boston: Kluwer Academic.

Ostrom, T. M., & Gannon, K. M. (1996). Exemplar generation: Assessing how respondents give meaning to rating scales. In N. Schwarz & S. Sudman (Eds.), *Answering questions: Methodology for determining cognitive and communicative processes in survey research.* San Francisco: Jossey-Bass.

Paul-Dauphin, A., Guillemin, F., et al. (1999). Bias and precision in visual analogue scales: A randomized controlled trial. *American Journal of Epidemiology, 150*(10), 1117–1127.

Pedhazur, E. J., & Schmelkin, L. P. (1991). *Measurement, design, and analysis: An integrated approach.* Mahwah, NJ: Erlbaum.

Pett, M. A., Lackey, N. R., & Sullivan, J. J. (2003). *Making sense of factor analysis: The use of factor analysis for instrument development in health care research.* Thousand Oaks, CA: Sage.

Popham, W. J. (1978). As always, provocative. *Journal of Educational Measurement, 15*(4), 297–300.

Preacher, K. J., & MacCallum, R. C. (2003). Repairing Tom Swift's electric factor analysis machine. *Understanding Statistics, 2*(1), 13-43.

Price, D. D., McGrath, P. A., et al. (1983). The validation of visual analogue scales as ratio scale measures for chronic and experimental pain. *Pain, 17*(1), 45–56.

Prochaska, J. O., & DiClemente, C. C. (1982). Transtheoretical therapy: Toward a more integrative model of change. *Psychotherapy: Theory, Research, and Practice, 19*(3), 276–287.

Rasch, G. (1960). *Studies in mathematical psychology I: Probabilistic models for some intelligence and attainment tests.* Copenhagen: Nielsen & Lydiche.

Rogers, E. M. (1995). *Diffusion of innovations.* New York: Free Press.

Rosenberg, M. (1965). *Society and the adolescent self-image.* Princeton, NJ: Princeton University Press.

Rosenberg, M. (1989). *Society and the adolescent self-image* (rev. ed.). Middletown, CT: Wesleyan University Press.

Rosenstock, I. M. (1960). What research in motivation suggests for public health. *American Journal of Public Health, 50,* 295–302.

Salant, P., & Dillman, D. (1994). *How to conduct your own survey.* New York: Wiley.

Schaeffer, N. C. (1991). Hardly ever or constantly? Group comparisons using vague quantifiers. *Public Opinion Quarterly, 55,* 395–423.

Schonlau, M., Fricker, R. D., & Elliott, M. N. (2002). *Conducting research surveys via e-mail and the web.* Santa Monica, CA: Rand.

Schuman, H., Presser, S., & Ludwig, J. (1981). Context effects on survey responses to questions about abortion. *Public Opinion Quarterly, 45*(2), 216–223.

Schwarz, N., et al. (1991). Rating scales: Numeric values may change the meaning of scale labels. *Public Opinion Quarterly, 55,* 570–582.

Schwarz, N., & Sudman, S. (1996). *Answering questions: Methodology for determining cognitive and communicative processes in survey research.* San Francisco: Jossey-Bass.

Shavelson, R. J., & Webb, N. M. (1991). *Generalizability theory: A primer.* Thousand Oaks, CA: Sage.

Silverman, I. (1977). *The human subject in the psychological laboratory.* New York: Pergamon Press.

Spearman, C. (1904). "General intelligence," objectively determined and measured. *American Journal of Psychology 15*(2), 201–293.

Spearman, C. (1910). Correlation calculated from faulty data. *British Journal of Psychology, 3,* 271–295.

Spector, P. E. (1992). *Summated rating scale construction: An introduction.* Thousand Oaks, CA: Sage.

SPSS. (2004). *SPSS 13.0 base user's guide.* Chicago: Author.

Stevens, S. S. (1946). On the theory of scales of measurement. *Science, 103,* 677–680.

Stevens, S. S. (1951). Mathematics, measurement and psychophysics. In *Handbook of experimental psychology* (pp. 1–49). New York: Wiley.

Stevens, S. S. (1959). Measurement, psychophysics and utility. In C. W. Churchman & P. Ratoosh (Eds.), *Measurement definitions and theories* (pp. 18–63). New York: Wiley.

Strack, R., Martin, L. L., et al. (1988). Priming and communication: Social determinants of information use in judgements of life-satisfaction. *European Journal of Social Psychology, 18,* 429–442.

Streiner, D. L., & Norman, G. R. (1995). *Health measurement scales: A practical guide to their development and use* (2nd ed.). New York: Oxford University Press.

Sudman, S. B., & Bradburn, N. M. (1982). *Asking questions.* San Francisco: Jossey-Bass.

Sudman, S., Bradburn, N. M., & Schwarz, N. (1996). *Thinking about answers: The application of cognitive processes to survey methodology.* San Francisco: Jossey-Bass.

Tabachnick, B. G., & Fidell, L. S. (2001). *Using multivariate statistics.* Boston: Allyn & Bacon.

Thorndike, E. L. (1913). *Educational psychology, Vol. II: The psychology of learning.* New York: Teachers College.

Thorndike, E. L. (1920). *Educational psychology.* New York: Teachers College.

Thurstone, L. L. (1925). A method of scaling psychological and educational tests. *Journal of Educational Psychology, 16*(7), 433–451.

Thurstone, L. L., & Chave, E. J. (1929). *The measurement of attitude: A psychophysical method and some experiments with a scale for measuring attitude toward the church.* Chicago: University of Chicago Press.

Tilden, V. P., Nelson, C. A., & May, B. A. (1990). The IPR inventory: Development and psychometric characteristics. *Nursing Research, 39*(6), 337–343.

Tourangeau, R., & Rasinski, K. (1988). Cognitive processes underlying context effects in attitude measurement. *Psychological Bulletin, 103*(3), 299–314.

Tourangeau, R., Rips, L. J., & Rasinski, K. (2000). *The psychology of survey response.* New York: Cambridge University Press.

Trochim, W. (2001). *The research methods knowledge base* (2nd ed.). Cincinnati: Atomic Dog.

Turner, R. C., & Carlson, L. (2003). Indexes of item-objective congruence for multidimensional items. *International Journal of Testing, 3*(2), 163–171.

Viswanathan, M. (2005). *Measurement error and research design.* Thousand Oaks, CA: Sage.

Walker, L. O., & Avant, K. C. (1988). *Strategies for theory construction in nursing* (2nd ed.). East Norwalk, CT: Appleton & Lang.

Waltz, C. F., Strickland, O. L., & Lenz, E. R. (1991). *Measurement in nursing research* (2nd ed.). Philadelphia: Davis.

Weinert, C. (2003). Measuring social support: PRQ2000. In O. L. Strickland & C. Di Iorio (Eds.), *Measurement of nursing outcomes* (pp. 161–172). New York: Springer.

Weiss, R. (1974). *The provision of social relationships. Doing unto others.* Upper Saddle River, NJ: Prentice-Hall.

Wilson, J. (1970). *Thinking with concepts.* New York, Cambridge University Press.

Wong, D. L., Hockenberry-Eaton, M., et al. (2001). *Wong's essentials of pediatric nursing* (6th ed.). St. Louis: Mosby.

Index

Printed and bound by CPI Group (UK) Ltd, Croydon, CR0 4YY

27/10/2024

14580323-0002